Existential Health Psychology

Patrick M. Whitehead

Existential Health Psychology

The Blind-spot in Healthcare

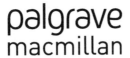

Patrick M. Whitehead
Sociology and Psychology
Albany State University
Albany, GA, USA

ISBN 978-3-030-21354-1   ISBN 978-3-030-21355-8   (eBook)
https://doi.org/10.1007/978-3-030-21355-8

Cover illustration: Pattern © John Rawsterne/patternhead.com

This Palgrave Pivot imprint is published by the registered company Springer Nature
Switzerland AG
The registered company address is: Gewerbestrasse 11, 6330 Cham, Switzerland

To my beautiful wife, Erica

FOREWORD

It is now fashionable to hear of one *existential crisis* or another. Seemingly out of nowhere the word existential is now regularly heard from the mouths of news entertainers, pundits, and politicians. One asserted that the planet has an expiration date of 2030, and with no edible food, no potable water, and no breathable air, soon after will follow the end of the existence of that most endangered subspecies of living things: *Homo sapiens sapiens*. We will no longer exist. Much like the aftermath of a nuclear holocaust, only cockroaches will remain.

My ears perk up, not because of the doomsday predictions, but because of the surprising resurrection of that word, which I thought had permanently disappeared with the post-World War II era I grew up in, along with avid readers of Walter Kaufmann's mélange of essays and excerpts from philosophy and literature *Existentialism from Dostoevsky to Sartre* and quirky plays such as *Waiting for Godot* or J.D. Salinger's *The Catcher in the Rye*, which captured the existential crisis of growing up better even than the ego psychobiographies of the ego psychologist Erik Erikson.

Beginning in the late 1940s, existentialism was a quasi-surrealist bit of Euroamerican intellectual exotica that remained in currency through the end of the 1960s. There had been several decades of talk about meaning and ultimate concerns as the planet recovered from World War II. People were enjoined to think, not just know and believe, and consider whether you ought to trust your perceptions over what you had learned. These were issues where psychology and philosophical considerations overlapped.

To speak of an existential threat to all human beings makes no sense, however. The existential pertains to the individual, not groups, let alone a subspecies or mineral item in the solar system. It refers to the situation of the singular, unique individual human being in a way that has nothing to do with what he is—his identity, self, ego, or personality. It is about existing, not being.

I suppose I am among the very few who actually welcome the return of the word existential after more than a half century, if only to question its usage. Its reappearance signals the uneasy consciousness of a sensibility that first produced the phenomenon of existentialism, when mankind was truly congealing globally and not just in the West and to where its influence had stretched. Every word bears a deeper history than people may be aware of, a point that the progenitor of existentialism had made beginning with his look at the vocabulary of early Greek thinking.

The word existence has disappeared from all but a few college psychology classrooms except mine. Even by 1972, when I taught my first undergraduate classes, while I continued to refer to Sartre, Maurice Merleau-Ponty, Jan van den Berg, Médard Boss, and Heidegger, my colleagues often ridiculed me. Students, however, were fascinated with what they heard and so I knew something was right. The way to understand us human beings, my colleagues insisted, was to examine the tissues of our brains and analyze the compounds they are soaked in and that circulate through our blood stream. If they were clinical psychologists, following on the ever more strident *DSM* trends in psychiatry after 1955 and the hegemony of the post-psychoanalytic world of behaviorism, they insisted students should focus exclusively on the observable behavior of specimens of creatures, from mice and rats, to college freshmen. In many places, the beginning psychologist studies hermit crabs to understand the principles of psychology. What *is* there, after all, except observable behavior?

The rules about what can be said about what *is* are broken, however, in the case of the being who raises the question about *being*: namely, the human being. Other beings do not raise the question or they do not need to: rocks, plants, birds, God. But we do—each of us—and that puts human beings in a unique, albeit highly problematic situation. To put as bluntly as possible: We never *are* something—we exist. Only when she dies can we say this existence, this *who*, is finally something, a what. Rocks, plants, birds, and God do not have to learn to be mineral, floral, avian, or divine. Humanity, however, is not there initially. It is conferred by another human being by way of an unfathomable alchemy and continues to be worked out through a lifetime: ever beginning, never finished. Its possibilities are inexhaustible no matter how constrained and limited the human being's environment may be—until the moment of death. Of course, these ideas were not new, but for the existentialists in the aftermath of the second "great" war they were vivid. And now, nearly a quarter of the way into the new century, we are again hearing of the existential. What's up?

Part of the initial disdain for existentialism followed the disregard of experience, which like consciousness was a notion as dead as William James, who had foregrounded the latter. Experience disappeared from the titles of introductory textbooks on psychology. Inner world and outer world were a black box and the environment, respectively, and since the lights never go on in the box, presumably we are left with what is out there for everyone to see—and only that—if we want to understand each other. But to understand just what, again? What about this being? The behaving organism was termed *l'homme machine*—man, the machine—as Julien Offray de la Mettrie had termed us in 1747, following on the astonishing claim made a century earlier by his fellow Frenchman, René Descartes, that animals below us in the taxonomy are nothing more than highly elaborate mechanisms, modeled on the clock. We are timekeeping living machines. Taught by Jesuits, however, Descartes had to find room in the human being for a soul. There it was, hidden away in a gland just north of the soft palate, but Mettrie eliminated the soul altogether. This most daring philosopher and physician (Descartes was "only" a philosopher), he had set the stage for the view of us—the wise, knowing creatures—that medical doctors following him would investigate as terribly complex mechanisms that had somehow come into view in the minds of certain men of science who in each case just happened to occupy such a machine. It is no coincidence that Mettrie was a physician and that, following him, the grounding disciplines of medicine today are chemistry and engineering—medicine as a science and a technology, for which being born, dying, wondering, feeling, imagining, and all the rest of "psychological life" is treated as discrete, albeit related biochemical events. Understandably, the darlings of science are artificial intelligence, cybernetics, and the robot.

Things changed in the twentieth century, however, when the science underlying psychology, Newtonian physics, was turned on its head and man the machine was (once again) found to be evil at times. In the Age of Enlightenment, we had evidently tried to forget that yet to be consistent evil must now also be explained biochemically. Alas, it belongs to a conceptually different universe than the cosmos comprising elements printed in the periodic table and ever cuter subatomic particles and weird forces tracked down every year. Between Mettrie and B.F. Skinner, Mary Shelley's hybrid of machine and organism, the monster dubbed "Beautiful" no less, had been envisioned. It should have been a warning, but instead it was turned into a movie and "he" has inspired a pantheon of superheroes. While the idea of a machine was elegant (and simple) like a clock, the monster was not. Like the human being "he" was designed to replicate, "he" was also spiritual, a *who*. The object of study of modern medical science had been invented.

With some presaging by the somewhat emotional mess and somewhat brilliant essayist of emotional life, Soren Kierkegaard, there finally came on the scene between the "war to end all wars" and its even more deadly version complete with nuclear bombs, the German thinker Martin Heidegger. His proposal, in 1927, that human being is of a sort that eludes the categories of every other sort of being (from rocks to God) that Aristotle, the philosopher who had great-great-great-...grandfathered science in his physics and metaphysics, was surprising. He described a unique set of "categories" called existentials that apply only to human beings in whom there is the unlikely, unpredictable confluence of animality, values, and a not so residual soul or spirit (*Geist*). In shock at what was happening in Europe, the French Heideggerian, Jean-Paul Sartre, seized on the master's subtlety, existence (*Da-sein*—literally, there-being), and translated it into something we human beings—good and evil alike—are responsible for, whether we wish it or not. There was a philosophical mistake in the translation, but *existence* was distilled in the retort of the alchemy of the French language and Existentialism as a form of humanism was born. Heidegger remained inaccessible to most intellectuals, but, in his plays and short stories, Sartre illustrated and brought to life a version of what Heidegger's "fundamental ontology" had attempted unsuccessfully to describe. In short, Sartre said, we may be machines, as Mettrie had said, but in the first place we exist. This means we are free and condemned to be free. The upshot was that being something or somebody and existing are not the same. Regardless of the misunderstanding, something important had been articulated and illuminated for two generations of professors. And now, once again, it is being named again. For us, existing is more fundamental than being.

It does not require an aptitude or taste for philosophy—from Aristotle to Sartre—or for psychology to understand what this brief history means for us now. It suffices instead to take some time to read Patrick Whitehead's new book on the medicalization of everyday life. Nowhere else than in the control of everyday life by medical warnings and remedies, interventions and technologies, is the echo of the message of the existentialists more evident. Among young psychology pedagogues we have in Whitehead someone who is exposing what it means to have made living a series of pathological conditions. The pervasiveness of modern medicine in every fold of skin and pore of the body social he reveals is striking. "The medical blind-spot misses the existential dimension of human being," he writes. Since medicine is everywhere, we have been blinded to what is essential—existence. In its hegemony, medicine has overpowered and dimmed down the uniqueness of the being that it claims to care for while doing it no harm. Recall *primum non nocere*: in the first place and above all, whatever else you do as a doctor, do no harm. This is the oath taken by every physician as a condition of being granted her license to practice this art.

As it turns out, while breathtaking interventions and achievements in surgery have given medicine a prestige that it well deserves, in having capitulated to seeing the organism as only a machine, physicians have become veterinarians for people, that most domesticated of all animals, and iatrogenic troubles have added to the woes of diseases that have plagued our subspecies from the start.

Professor Whitehead is as familiar with Martin Heidegger as with Kurt Goldstein, with Wilhelm Wundt and William James as with Thomas Szasz. The reader—especially the young reader—will benefit by being (re)introduced to these important thinkers. Whitehead understands that the history of medicine and psychology did not begin in 1980 or soon after, and that both have underlying philosophical and ideological agendas that those who teach and practice in both disciplines must understand. There is no presuppositionless philosophy, and all of modern science, including medicine and psychology, are based on a philosophical position that must be honestly acknowledged.

This is also an important book for reintroducing some figures who first brought the existential dimension into psychology, including Médard Boss and R.D. Laing. Both were properly trained physicians and psychiatrists, but influenced by existentialism, they offered the shocking possibility that there might be something unusual, if not special, about *Homo sapiens sapiens*: it exists. The reader is brought to look back before looking forward in order to understand that a *who* is not a *what*. Whitehead is worried (as I am) to see that love, sadness, and enthusiasm, for example, have disappeared in the current mythology (I might even say religion) of neurotransmitters and biochemical reactions. There is no place for action and freedom in a world explained *entirely* in terms of reactions.

The present volume encourages us to pause when we hear that the brain decides or prefers something, wishes or hates somebody. Tissues do not feel and speak, parts of the brain do not communicate with each other like the first on-line chatters, Alexander Graham Bell and his assistant, Thomas Watson. Yet most viewers of commercials for psychotropic medications are supposed to believe this. It was not long ago that people believed in the power of ghosts and demons to determine behavior, or that the shape of one's skull or the color of one's skin compelled them to act in certain ways without redemption. We are now supposed to believe in chemicals with appetites, needs, and desires. This is not a book that dismisses science or rejects the remarkable accomplishments of modern medicine but simply warns that the focus of a doctor's practice must first and always be the existing human being and not a living version of the corpse he dissected in medical school. It will be difficult for some readers to suspend certain beliefs they cherished that are disguised as knowledge. But they should try.

We have been mistaken in speaking of medicine as health care. It is illness care. At its best, medicine is care for the existence of a human being whose temporary passive patient status calls first for a human response—the response of another existing human being—followed by whatever interventions may be cautiously made providing that no harm is done. Having become blind to the patient's existence, medicine now does harms. It remains to be seen how extensive the influence of Whitehead's book will be, but it requires our attention.

Wagner College   Miles Groth
New York, NY, USA
March 27, 2019

ACKNOWLEDGMENTS

This book would not have been possible without the support of my university, Albany State University. Dorene Medlin and the Center for Faculty of Excellence helped finance a trip for me to present an early version of "Existential Health Psychology" at an APA conference in Boulder, CO, and she also helped organize a community presentation here in Albany. Special thanks are also due to Hema Mason, my department chair, whose support of faculty scholarship goes well above and beyond her administrative duties. I would also like to thank my students—many of them on their way to becoming nurses, anesthetists, and physical or occupational therapists—whose interest in the topics of health and well-being have directed my own scholarship over the past few years.

I am, of course, also indebted to the work of those who came before me, laying the pathway toward a more human practice of medicine. Most notably, this includes Kurt Goldstein, Martin Heidegger, Médard Boss, Ivan Illich, and Arthur Kleinman. The names of additional scholars also line the pages that follow. More recently, I have benefited tremendously from the scholarship, consultation, and support of Miles Groth and Kevin Aho. Thank you both for your help.

Thank you to Rachel and Madison at Palgrave who have worked with me to navigate the review, contract, and editorial processes and to help produce a quality finished piece. Thank you as well to the anonymous peer reviewers whose support and recommendation made its selection possible.

Finally, I would like to thank my beautiful wife, Erica, who is herself an internal medicine specialist. Thank you for your patience in putting up with my fascination and concern with medicine, especially when it so often challenges the routines and procedures that comprise your professional world. Thank you for the stories about your patients, many of which can be found in anecdotes across a few of the chapters. Thank you for your support in my writing, and my career more generally. I love you.

Two of these chapters have been presented previously. Chapter 6 was presented at the 2018 Division 32 APA mid-Winter meeting as "Existential Health Psychology: What It Is and Isn't" in February of 2018, and the concluding chapter was presented as a public lecture at Albany State University as "The Blindspot in Healthcare" in September of 2018.

Contents

CHAPTER 1

Introduction: The Blind-spot in Medicine

Abstract An introduction to the blind-spot in medicine: human existence is systematically left out of healthcare. Two stories are told that introduce this blind-spot. The first is that of Kurt Goldstein, the World War I German neuropsychiatrist who describes a crisis in modern medicine. The second is that of Médard Boss, a World War II Swiss neuropsychiatrist who finds that medicine has trained him poorly to treat problems of meaning and existence. Time is spent differentiating existential health psychology from health psychology and complementary or alternative medical models.

Keywords Kurt Goldstein • Médard Boss • Martin Heidegger • Modern medicine • Health psychology

Humans have an ocular blind-spot in each eye. The neurobiologists explain the ocular blind-spot phenomenon by describing how there are no light-sensitive neurons on the retina where the optic nerve exits at the rear of the eye, and therefore no sense data can be processed there. This is actually a pretty good way for describing how a splotch might appear on the screen of your smartphone: an absence of photon-producing pixels.

Even after many years of teaching sensation and perception to college students, I am still surprised to learn that many are reluctant to accept that they have a blind-spot in their visual field. The reason why the visual blind-spot is seldom recognized is that they have never had any reason to perceive it.

P. M. Whitehead, *Existential Health Psychology*,
https://doi.org/10.1007/978-3-030-21355-8_1

Indeed, it seems that it is only useful as a gimmick in the general psychology classroom. Far more interesting than the fact of our blind-spot is that the latter is routinely ignored.

If you have ever used a smartphone with a cracked screen, or driven a car with a cracked windshield, you will remember how distracting the crack was initially. You had grown accustomed to a particular interaction between yourself and your smartphone (or car), and now this crack has inserted itself into this routine. Eventually, you learn to navigate the miniature, backlit, rectangular world of search engines, GIFs, and videos despite the visual impediment. The impediment fades away from your awareness, and you eventually stop noticing it.

Sunglasses tint the light in your spectral world only until you have grown accustomed to the tint—then you might even forget that you are wearing sunglasses at all. You adapt to a new routine—a new way of making sense of the world and of understanding your interactions within it.

These kinds of blind-spots can be understood by the phenomenon of sensory accommodation. This occurs when something is present and available to your perception in a continuous way—be it a smell, sound, or tactile sensation. While it is noticed at first, after a while it begins to fade away. A hospital room, for example, might initially smell funny, have a distracting number of whirrs and beeps, and be dimly lit. These are all noticeable at first, but after a while they fade away. It is not that they have disappeared, but you no longer actively discriminate between them in your perception. If, for example, the beeping was to stop, then you would probably notice that something had changed even if you could not quite identify what it was. Sensory blindness due to accommodation occurs *when the meaning of the perceptions* (such as the funny smell in the hospital room) *is insignificant.*

Sometimes, however, blind-spots contain information that is very significant: such as those that occur as a consequence of your position within your car and its position on the road. Seated in the driver's seat, you have an excellent view of the direction you are heading. A sprawling windshield allows you to see nearly everything in front of the car. Three mirrors capture views in the reverse—rear, right-rear, and left-rear. Even with these four perspectives combined, there are a few views that are missed entirely—views that can be large enough to fit a minivan full of children. Unless you are diligent enough as a driver to look over your shoulder to examine this vehicular blind-spot, there is no way of knowing what is being missed.

Checking blind-spots while driving isn't just a helpful practice, it is essential. To be sure, it is uncommon to be *surprised* by what you find when you do. But even if you are surprised only once out of 100 (or 1000) times, the practice of checking will have been worth it.

I have described two kinds of blind-spots above. The first can be understood through sensory accommodation, which happens when the meaning of a particular perception proves insignificant. The second has to do with the way a practice or procedure has been designed. The structure, seating, and setup of the contemporary automobile (as well as the infrastructure of the road and highway systems) make vehicular blind-spots a reality. Engineering can go into minimizing the visibility limitations, such as with the development of rear and side-view cameras, but unless roads prohibit any kind of driving that is not single file, there will always be the risk of blind-spot under-sight.

Modern medicine has a blind-spot. Like the vehicular blind-spot, it is enormously significant. Also like the vehicular blind-spot, the medical blind-spot is also a consequence of the way that medicine has been developed. Like side-viewing cameras on automobiles, it wouldn't take an enormous change to notice the medical blind-spot. However, medicine has been practicing with this blind-spot for so long that it has become increasingly difficult to *notice* what is being left out. It amounts to trying to get college students to discover their visual blind-spot. Some students are eager to see it and understand—"how will I know when I have found it?" While others fold their arms indignantly—"I don't have one; nobody has one; this is ridiculous."

The medical blind-spot also shares something in common with the blind-spot of sensory accommodation. With the latter, we no longer notice something because it has proven insignificant: we have not had to understand the world by way of this phenomenological detail so it fades away. With the medical blind-spot, a particular way of viewing health, wellness, and the practice of medicine has resulted in ignoring additional aspects of health and wellness.[1] *Because* the latter are systematically ignored, they are understood to be insignificant. Finally, because they are understood to be significant, they have faded from view.

The medical blind-spot misses the existential dimension of human being—the structure of meaning through which experiences always unfold. This obviously doesn't happen over the course of a year or even a

---

[1] Particularly those that are existential in nature or that pertain specifically to being that humans are.

decade. It takes *many* decades. The modern iteration of medicine did not begin by neglecting its existential dimension. The latter was merely an effect of viewing the medical subject scientifically. Moreover, the experimental handling of medicine has experienced many decades of improvements (which will be explored further in Chap. 4). As generations of providers were trained within the medical model, with no mention of the existential dimension of health and wellness, it became easy to assume that the latter was insignificant. Indeed, even the language surrounding it has come to seem awkward and unhelpful.

To trace the historical development of the medical blind-spot, I will begin by going back 100 years to World War I, when German neuropsychiatrist Kurt Goldstein was noticing that the medical model had left out an essential ingredient to the understanding of health and wellness. For Goldstein, the blind-spot concerned the meaningful coherence of organic activity—a phenomenon he called self-actualization. Goldstein notices the blind-spot as an effect of the scientific practice of medicine and warns fellow providers not to get stuck within any particular (but limiting) paradigm of medical practice. Next, I will move the clock forward 25 years to World War II, where a Swiss psychiatrist, Médard Boss, was realizing that something was being left out of modern medical practice. By then, the problem was becoming more and more difficult to articulate. At a loss for words, Boss consults with German existential phenomenological philosopher Martin Heidegger, eventually asking him to come to his clinic to teach the other resident physicians.

Kurt Goldstein Identifies a Crisis in Medicine

As a German neuropsychiatrist during World War I, Kurt Goldstein was assigned to work with soldiers who had suffered closed-head injuries. In the early part of the twentieth century, neuropsychology and psychiatry had not yet been established the way that they are today. Indeed, the first neuropsychiatric department of a hospital was not developed in the United States until the 1920s at Harvard, under the direction of Karl Lashley. The lack of research into and protocol for handling closed-head injuries made the work of neuropsychiatrists during World War I exceedingly important, and few would become more influential than Goldstein.[2]

---

[2] His influence is even more impressive when it is understood that Goldstein, as a Jewish physician, was denied professorships at major German universities and even arrested while

When applied to closed-head injuries, the model of modern medicine suggests that deficits in behavior or cognition could be explained by deficits in the brain, even when the brain could not be seen directly. If a soldier is admitted with paralysis of his right arm, then it could be concluded that the "right-arm-area" of the primary motor cortex had been damaged. At the time, this method was called associationism (but it is now called the identity hypothesis). Associationism is the assumption that discrete brain regions are responsible for discrete cognitive and behavioral functions. If the "right-arm-area" of my brain is damaged, then I cannot rehabilitate right-hand activities and must instead learn to go about my duties without it. If, however, I had merely torn a rotator cuff, then I could be prescribed a series of stretching and strengthening practices in order to rehabilitate full right-arm mobility.

Goldstein's assignment was to determine who was injured and who was malingering. Of those who were injured, he was to determine who could be rehabilitated (to return to battle) and who must be discharged. To do so, his task was to identify the presenting symptoms and trace these to the nervous system in order to determine what neurological damage had been done. Here's how it should have gone: (1) identify the behavioral deficits (deficit *a*, deficit *b*, etc.); (2) determine the locus of the deficits (locus *a*, locus *b*, etc.); (3) prescribe rehabilitation plan, if any.

This presents an easy-to-follow guide for understanding the newly emerging field of neuropsychiatry. It follows exactly the steps of any other diagnostic-prognostic strategy in modern medicine, whether one has found a broken leg or lung infection. Record the symptoms; identify the underlying cause of the symptoms; focus treatment on the underlying cause. This is what you attempt to do when you search for your symptoms on WebMD or Wikipedia. You compare the symptoms associated with a whole bunch of discovered diseases and compare them to your own, then follow the recommended courses of treatment.

When trying to follow this 1-2-3 method, Goldstein quickly found that there was an impossible feature in the first step. The first step, you will recall, deals with the determination of symptoms. Evidently, there are many problems that accompany this step. The title of Section I, Chapter 1 of *The Organism* captures this: "The Problem of the Determination of Symptoms." In this section, chapter, and throughout the book, Goldstein

seeing patients. He spent a year in jail before it was arranged for him to emigrate to the United States, which he admits never quite felt like home.

lists many problems with the symptom focus, beginning with how to determine which symptom is the important one. One problem with the symptom-determination approach that Goldstein observes is that a symptom can never be isolated to one aspect of the patient's behavior. For example, a tear in the plantar fascia is not *only* evident when the fascia must contract but may be seen in the global modification of the patient's behavior—like a reluctance to put weight on that leg, or a refusal to stand. From where, then, do these symptoms emanate?

The Organism is full of such observations that Goldstein has about the then-novel modern medical approach. He operates within these discourses to a certain degree, as they had become the dominant medical discourses of that time. To this end, he writes the following of the symptom-determination, diagnosis, prognosis method: "The fundamental principle of this procedure is, of course, reasonable" (p. 34).

For Goldstein, alternatives to this always seemed just around another corner, and he was able to weave discussions of neurological and existential trauma together without contradictions or impasses. He was able to see *and* describe the shortcomings of the modern medical approach as it pertained to the treatment of closed-head injuries. He also recognized the danger of assuming that the modern medical model has the answers to all medical questions. To this end, he issues a powerful warning regarding the medical trend that was becoming increasingly dominant:

> The real crisis arises when, even in the face of new findings, the investigator cannot free himself from the former theory; rather, the scientist attempts to preserve it and, by constant emendations, to reconcile it with these new facts instead of replacing it by a new theory fitted to deal with both the old and new facts. This error has not been avoided in the evolution of the classical doctrine. (p. 35)

MÉDARD BOSS PUZZLES OVER LANGUAGE TO DESCRIBE TIME, BEING

As an able-bodied Swiss man in the 1940s, psychiatrist Médard Boss was enlisted for service in the military as a battalion doctor. With the provision of a handful of hard working doctors who reported directly to him, Boss found himself gripped with boredom during his tour of duty (it was Switzerland, after all). His newfound boredom led to a growing preoccupation with the concept of time, which had suddenly become a problem for him.

The phenomenon of boredom is an interesting one. It seems as though one is oppressed by something from without—as if some *thing* has robbed one's activities of purpose, direction, and meaning. Neuropsychologists might search for the brain region that is responsible for the desirability of going for a walk or mixing a vodka martini while psychoanalysts might suggest that one's psyche or ego is being smothered by something—a past memory, trauma, or Other (person). In order to be a phenomenon in modern medicine, boredom must be some*thing*. More specifically, something that causes the familiar behavioral and motivational changes in you and me.

Of course, none of these are quite right. I do not *have* an ego or self to be oppressed any more than my brain can *feel* desire[3] (or lack thereof). What, then, was Boss to make of this newfound sense of boredom?

It was upon this backdrop that Boss came across a news item about a book titled *Being and Time* written by German philosopher Martin Heidegger. He ordered a copy and began reading. In *Being and Time* (*Sein und Zeit*, published in 1927), Heidegger attempts a fundamental ontology. Instead of building up "human being" by adding together blocks of chemical elements and carbon chains, the way that modern science has sought to understand the human body, Heidegger carefully described the foundation of human *being*.

Heidegger's work begins with by rejecting the idea that everybody *already knows* what Being is. Contrary to modern thinking, Heidegger maintained that "human being" and "existence" are not merely the activities of an objectified body. This is the natural conclusion that must be drawn when following the steps of the scientific method, but it leaves something important out: namely, what *being* means. Heidegger (1962) explains: "So if it is said that 'Being' is the most universal concept, this cannot mean that it is the one which is clearest or that it needs no further discussion. It is rather the darkest of all" (p. 23).

Too briefly, human *being* (which is a gerund—an action word in the present) is translated by modern science into its past state (i.e., having been). Science cannot capture skiing, but can identify one who skis; it can-

---

[3] Unfortunately, the latter position has become a typical one among psychologists and philosophers alike. An example of the growing popularity of the-brain-that-feels can be seen in the publication of *Neuroexistentialism* (Caruso and Flanagan 2018), where a broad mixture of authors discuss how the very existential I describe is being left out of medicine may be found in the nervous system.

not capture mothering, but it can identify one who mothers. Being is always replaced with having been. Living beings are replaced with lifeless bodies. Boredom cannot be understood as a past-state thing, but only a present engagement in the world: only as an action.

Boss quickly learned that his training in biomedical science had not prepared him to understand Heidegger's rendering of human existence—*Dasein*. *Dasein*, which may be translated into English as "being there," is the quality of being that is unique to humans (at least from the perspective of humans). It is the quality of existing. For Heidegger, time is not a taken-for-granted dimension of physical universe, but an opening, a space, or a possibility of becoming. As such, it is not a physical dimension, but an existential one.

Thoroughly confused by what he had read, Boss eventually built up the courage to correspond directly with the philosopher himself. This began over a decade of correspondence between the two. When he realized the value of Heidegger's philosophy for his own practice of medicine, Boss organized a seminar format for interested physicians. They met initially at the Burgholzie Hospital, which eventually changed to Boss's own house in Zollikon, Sweden, for ten years between 1959 and 1969. The lectures and subsequent conversations were documented in the book *Zollikon Seminars: Protocols—Conversations—Letters*. These will be described further in Chap. 4.

The important development with this story was how Boss was incapable not only of finding the words to describe the limitations he had experienced with medicine, but also of understanding the words once they had been presented to him. Only 25 years had passed from the caution that Goldstein had given to physicians regarding the problematic limitations imposed by the modern medical model, and the latter had already snuffed out the meaning of injury and illness that Goldstein had described.

As Boss eventually became more acquainted with the existentially oriented language of Heidegger, he began to realize that his colleagues would also benefit from these conversations. This is how the Zollikon Seminars came to be. Like Boss, the Zollikon physicians struggled and fumbled through their attempts to even describe human being, always instead trying to discuss it in terms of past states—as objects of modern science. Consider, for example, the following exchange:

Martin Heidegger: ...how does bodiliness [embodiment[4]], which is unde-termined, relate to space?

    Seminar Participant: The body is nearest to us in space.

    MH: I would say that it is the most distant. ... Because you are educated in anatomy and physiology as doctors, that is, with a focus on the examina-tion of bodies, you probably look at the states of the body in a different way than the "layman" does. Yet, a layman's experience is probably closer to the phenomenon of pain as it involves our body lines, even if it can hardly be described with the aid of our usual intuition of space. (pp. 83–84)

Notice how Heidegger suggests these physicians might have to first *unlearn* their own unique way of viewing the inert body of medicine in order to understand the body existentially. By the 1960s, the medical dis-courses had neglected the layman's experience of suffering for so long that it became impossible to consider it at all. Patient suffering had become irrelevant to medicine.

The seminars are full of exchanges where Heidegger asks the physicians to unlearn the medical perspective. He develops lines of reasoning that seem counterintuitive to the modern scientific mindset. "Being cannot be glimpsed by science" (2001, p. 18).

When Goldstein attempted to understand his patients using the meth-ods of modern science, he realized that a great deal had been left out. Hundred years ago, he was able to describe the blind-spot of medicine, indicating its shortcomings and advancing postulates that would address them. At that time, there was still a language for expressing these concerns and a medical audience who understood.

Twenty-five years later, and through the 1960s, we find how Boss and his colleagues similarly realized that something had been left out. This time, however, they were not quite sure what that something might be or how it could best be articulated. The medical blind-spot had been formed. There was no longer any meaningful language left with which to describe it.

The medical blind-spot is with respect to human *being*—that which is uniquely human. This is particularly unfortunate since medicine is in ser-vice to human *being*, and not just their bodies. It is as Boss describes it in

---

[4] Embodiment is the existential dimension that includes the body. You and I do not *have* bodies; we *are* embodied. Our interactions with one another and with the world can only come by way of our bodies. The body does not bump into physical things and initiate a series of neurochemical impulses that terminate at our "minds." Our bodies are our capacity for interaction.

his 1970 publication of *Existenzgrundlage von Medizin und Psychologie* (*Existential Foundation of Medicine and Psychology*[5]):

> Assuming that the true subject matter of medicine is man, the whole reality of day-to-day human existence, we shall learn from our study that the natural scientific approach repeatedly finds itself confronting a realm to which it cannot gain access. It is precisely the essence of the way people behave among themselves in their daily lives, how they conduct themselves toward the world and other creatures, that modern medicine's natural scientific research method fails even to approach, much less to clarify in its uniqueness. (1979, p. xxviii)

For Boss, the medical blind-spot (human existence) is very much a part of medicine. Unfortunately, the latter has become less and less accommodating of the former. It seems that today, human existence can only be addressed within a new medical sub-discipline—that of existential medicine (Aho 2018) or, what would amount to the same thing, existential health psychology, as these share the same existential foundation.

Existential Medicine Is Not Complementary, Alternative, or Holistic

When discussing my work with medical providers, I have been asked about its relationship with complementary and alternative approaches to medicine (CAM), as well as with holistic medicine. This has been frequent enough to require brief attention at the outset. Existential medicine and existential health psychology are not synonymous with these other approaches to medicine and health, and they should not be confused.

To be sure, you will find overlap between existential medicine, CAM, and holistic medicine, but not enough to justify their conflation. CAM includes those interventions that are rooted in historical, spiritual, indigenous, and regional traditions. Traditional practices—folk medicine, spiritual healing, herbal supplements, and changes to diet—go back millennia. Every culture has its own set of techniques for raising children, handling

---

[5] The original German title preserves Boss's recognition that medicine and psychology shared the same existential foundation. There is not an existential psychology (focusing, e.g., on the "psyche") that is distinct from the existential foundation of medicine (focusing, e.g., on the body). When it was translated into English.

conflict, and treating illnesses. As they have been lumped together into the category of CAM, these traditions have become medicalized—goods to be presided over by specialists and consumed by prospective patients. These have recently been subjected to the same kind of randomized medical trials that are the hallmark of experiment-based modern medicine. Herbal remedies, acupuncture, and energy healing, along with hundreds of others, have been subjected to placebo-controlled clinical trials in order to measure their precise therapeutic efficacy.

So too with holistic medicine. Aaron Antonovsky's "salutogenenic model," which will be described in more detail in Chap. 2, is a helpful example of holistic medicine. Antonovsky is careful to emphasize that health is not merely concerned with the biochemistry of the human body, but also includes aspects of lifestyle that have customarily been left out of the medical discussions—nutrition, finances, relationships, and so forth. While his data was primarily qualitative, the many aspects of health he has indicated have been individually subjected to massive clinical trials in order to determine their precise role in the mediation of health and wellness with chronic diseases. This is why you may have heard that your personal relationships influence your health, or that certain amounts of exercise and limited portions of potato chips can be helpful in "increasing" your health.

Existential medicine and existential health psychology belong to a conversation that does not include measurement, control, or any other objectification of human being and existence. It begins with the latter, specifically in cases of illness where a person's life and/or health has become a problem for them. These are not symptoms which are allegedly discrete, verifiable, and measurable. They are changes to one's way of being—one's routines in life.

Modern medicine, CAM, and holistic medicine are each tasked with intervention: intervening on behalf of the sick, ill, or diseased person in order to help them overcome their suffering. Existential medicine and health psychology target a non-objectifying understanding of the suffering (and existence) so that it may be accepted, and growth may continue.

Finally, and since we are on the subject, it is also important to note that you might also find overlap between existential medicine and conventional medicine. Conventional medicine has also come to include the growing field of health psychology, represented by Division 38 of the American Psychological Association. The mission of Division 38 specifies biomedicine as the preferable model of health. In the cases where overlap occurs, it is usually because the provider has left behind the strictures of modern science, departing from the evidence-based practices and procedures. At such times, it is understood that they are stepping outside of their roles as doctors, nurses, and clinicians and they are having human interactions. The human interactions are not credentialed, certified, or otherwise mediated by the state- and federally regulated medical institutions, and are therefore not "medical." Fortunately, with the work of figures such as Rita Charon (2018), Arthur Kleinman (1988), and Janice Morse (2016), there is a growing body of healthcare research that may be found stepping just outside of the modern medical model.

REFERENCES

Aho, K. (2018). Existential medicine: Heidegger and the lessons from Zollikon. In K. Aho (Ed.), *Existential medicine* (pp. xi–xxiv). Lanham: Rowman & Littlefield.

Boss, M. (1979). *Existential foundations of medicine and psychology* (S. Conway & A. Cleaves, Trans.). New York: Jason Aronson.

Caruso, G. D., & Flanagan, O. (2018). *Neuroexistentialism: Meaning, morals, & purpose in the age of neuroscience.* Cambridge, MA: Harvard University Press.

Charon, R. (2018). *Keynote address.* Washington, DC: National Endowment of the Humanities.

Heidegger, M. (2001). *Zollikon seminars: Protocols—Conversations—Letters* (M. Boss, Ed., and F. Mayr & R. Askay, Trans.). Evanston: Northwestern University Press.

Heidegger, M. (2008). *Being and time* (J. Macquarrie & E. Robinson, Trans.). New York: Harper Perennial. (Original translation published in 1962).

Kleinman, A. (1988). *Illness narratives: Suffering, healing, and the human condition.* New York: Basic Books.

Morse, J. (2016). *Qualitative health research: Creating a new discipline.* New York: Routledge.

CHAPTER 2

A History of Medical Care

Abstract This chapter describes the history of modern medicine and the growth in popularity of medical science. This requires a description of the experimental scientific foundations of medical science. Next, the successes and shortcomings of the biomedical model, that is, the disease- or pathology model of illness, are explored. This is followed by a description of holistic medicine, specifically the salutogenic model of Aaron Antonovsky. It is maintained that both pathogenic and salutogenic models of health miss the blind-spot described in the introduction.

Keywords Pathogenesis • History of medicine • Salutogenesis • Holistic biology

Modernity brought with it a number of changes to the lifestyles enjoyed in the West. This includes transportation, water treatment, plumbing, printing, and a wealth of other technologies. For example, travel by train, plane, and automobile is added to ship travel as a method for getting around, changing the social geography of the world. Cities used to develop around major ports, which is why New York, New Orleans, and the many stops along the Hudson and Mississippi rivers grew so quickly in the United States. Once the trans-continental train system was developed, cities where major connections occurred began to dictate growth, such as with Cincinnati or Atlanta.

© The Author(s) 2019
P. M. Whitehead, *Existential Health Psychology*,
https://doi.org/10.1007/978-3-030-21355-8_2

The practice of medicine has also seen a great transformation at the hands of modernity. Before the modern scientific practice of medicine, there were a number of medical theories that were practiced over time. Humorism, practiced by the ancient Greeks, is based on the idea of balance, centeredness, and equilibrium. These are familiar terms in medicine even today. But instead of balancing diet, lifestyle, and exercise, humorists balanced the four humors which were understood to regulate the human body: black bile, yellow bile, phlegm, and blood. With humorism, the healthy individual was the one in whom these four humors were in balance. Illnesses, diseases, and pain were understood as one of these four being out of balance. For example, a common practice was bloodletting (draining the blood out of a diseased person)—a practice that later would no longer receive the endorsement from medicine.

Through a series of chance discoveries and dedicated experimental findings, the modern practice of medicine has evolved over the last three centuries. An infection that would have resulted in death 100 years ago requires only an oral medication and a few days' rest today. Pneumonia, an infection now routinely diagnosed and treated, was the leading cause of death in the United States in the early twentieth century (1900s). Infant mortality (i.e., the percentage of children who die before the age of one) has been cut in half three times since the middle of the nineteenth century (from 41% in 1860 to 5% in 2015; Roser 2018[1]).

THE PRACTICE OF MODERN MEDICINE: THE PATHOGENIC MODEL

The success of Modern Medicine may be traced to the implementation of the pathogenic model of disease. This has allowed medical practice to benefit from the rigor and control of experimentation.

Before describing the pathogenic model of illness, a few words must first be said about the practice of modern science. The practice of experimentation officially begins in the seventeenth century with physicists Newton and Galileo. Experimentation is the process of making systematic observations of objects in the world and their relationships with other objects, and then testing these relationships. We can only understand a rock once we have subjected it to a number of procedures, testing its various properties. Hardness is not a property that belongs to the rock, but

[1] https://ourworldindata.org/child-mortality

one that belongs to the relationship between the rock and other solid objects. You determine which material is hardest by performing a scratch test: rub the two objects together and see which scratches the other. With experimentation, one does not merely conclude that a given rock is hard but compares its hardness with an array of other objects in order to specify precisely how hard the rock is with respect to these others.

Another important element of experimentation is *empiricism*—the use of observation by way of the five human senses. In order for you and I to observe something, that something has to be *observable*. If I cannot see, hear, feel, smell, or taste something, then I cannot be certain that it exists at all. In order to conduct experiments, scientists must rely on their senses in order to make observations about the world. Because the practice of experimentation requires observability, the latter has become synonymous with *real*.

To the modern scientist, observability does not count if it cannot be corroborated by another. This means that reality must also have the quality of publicity. If I find the temperature in the classroom to be cold, but everybody else finds it to be warm, then my perception—even though it has come by way of tactile perception—cannot be understood as a public one. It would instead have the quality of privacy: available only to me. Though it is my experience, it is not understood to be *real* the way that the thermometer publicly measures temperature. Instead of my private perception of cold and your private perception of hot, we may refer to the dash-mark to which the mercury spreads within the glass thermometer tube. The thermometer tube is public and verifiable to others. It is in this way that you and I can come to some agreement regarding the *real* temperature in the classroom.

When it is measured in this way, temperature is the relationship that mercury has with its immediate environment. You and I do not feel this mercury expanse. While our skin expands in the heat and contracts in the cold, it does not stretch out with the measurable ease as does the mercury in its glass tube. Our experience of temperature is fundamentally different from the interaction of mercury and temperature. However, we begin to understand our own experience of temperature by way of the thermometer. As it is measured by a thermometer, it is heat in its objectivity. Increasingly, this has come to be understood as *real* heat.

When we put publicity and systematic empiricism together with the idea that objects in the universe have distinct properties that can be understood, we arrive at objectivity: the model of modern science. Within this model, things are understood to be *real* only insofar as they have these objective properties. It is important to keep in mind that we cannot directly experience the world in its objectivity. We can only experience it empirically (through our direct experience). You and I can experience something as the sun sets over Lake Michigan, but unless that something can be evaluated objectively, then we can doubt whether or not the qualities of our experience were real.

These are interesting to reconcile with some of the myths and stories we tell—even when the stories are works of fiction. For example, in ghost stories, ghosts always have publicly observable qualities and are associated with changes in temperatures felt through the skin, apparitions captured by the eye, or sounds gathered by the ears (evidently, tasting or smelling a ghost has proven too intimate). In order for ghosts to be real, they must somehow register on our objective modes of observation. Never mind the traditional practices of sitting with, celebrating, visiting, or seeking counsel from the dead.

The practice of modern medicine has taken the quality of objectivity to be central. Therefore, the first step in treating an infection or disease is in seeing, feeling, hearing, tasting, or smelling the infection or disease. A patient is not treated for a cough, runny nose, or chest pain, because these are empirically ambiguous, first-person descriptions. Pneumonia, for example, can be experienced as a shortness of breath, coughing, and stabbing pain in the chest, but it cannot be diagnosed this way. It can only be diagnosed in its objectivity. Before it has been so diagnosed, the pneumonia is not yet real.

Because of the necessity of empirical observability, diseases are *discovered*. This is not unlike how chemists discover new chemical compounds or explorers have discovered new lands. Once a disease has manifested and has been documented, it may be searched for within the affected biochemistry of the ill person. Once *found*, treatment can commence.

Another important element of experimentation is control: in order to understand the qualities of a particular variable (such as an elevated body temperature), all other variables must be controlled (such as dehydration, ambient temperature, and so forth). If all other variables are controlled, then it can be concluded that an observation has been made about the variable in question and has not been mistaken for something else.

Modern medicine has effectively implemented these qualities of scientific experimentation into medical practice. As late as the nineteenth century (a scant 120 years ago), infectious diseases were the leading causes of death. Today, they have fallen nearly off the chart of expected causes of death. Last year more people died driving on the interstate than of viral infection in the United States. This means that the modern medical model has been exceedingly helpful in minimizing—nearly eradicating—what were once the leading causes of death.

However, the effectiveness of modern medicine has only been demonstrated in the treatment of pathogens. A pathogen can be understood as a foreign invader—a substance in the body that has impaired the latter's functioning. It is a thing that must be located, isolated, and treated. Medications are engineered to accomplish what seems like a direct attack on the invading pathogen. The practice of medicine is viewed as a medical battle between the patriotic doctors and the foreigner invaders—the bacterium, virus, or what have you. But they don't exactly work in this manner. For example, antibiotics help boost the immune system while anti-inflammatories and fever reducers help manage symptoms. Neither of these attack pathogens but allow bodily equilibrium to restore itself.

The pathogenic model of medicine is fashioned after a battle between good and evil. Health, the products of medicine, and medical providers are good, while any form of suffering is evil. Moreover, like influenza, it is assumed in advance that suffering can be treated. But as I have pointed out, influenza is not attacked by flu medication. Flu medication helps manage symptoms while the illness runs its course and bodily equilibrium is restored. This pales in comparison to the idea that medical science is the antidote to suffering and that suffering is ultimately preventable. The battle being waged, and the role of beneficent medical specialists in this, is part of the pathogenic medical narrative in which we all participate.

The pathogenic model also has the benefit of what French philosopher and physician Georges Canguilhem (1991) has called an ontological representation. The pathogen, which is understood to be the cause of suffering, legitimizes the suffering and makes it real. When afflicted with the common cold, complete with nasal congestion, sore throat, and lethargy, I do not yet have a medical condition. My experience is one of difficulty feeling energized to handle my daily routine, discomfort trying to sleep, a more sonorous than usual speaking voice, and an unquenchable thirst. These are transformations of how I feel and who I am. These changes occur across my personality. As such, the effect is difficult to circumscribe in a simple manner. However, within the pathogenic model, all of these may be understood as symptoms of an underlying pathogen. While I may take a medication to make it easier to fall asleep, the understanding is that

I am treating the virus associated with the common cold: I *have* the common cold—a pathogen that has rooted itself within my nasal passage, chest, and bowels, as it were.

In each case of disorder or disease, it is understood that there is a pathogen-thing at the source of the affliction to which the many experiential transformations can be attributed. Indeed, the very presence of the pathogen-thing is what validates the reality of the disorder or disease. Canguilhem explains: "Parkinson's disease is more of a disease than thoracic shingles, which is, in turn, more so than boils" (p. 39). He continues,

> the germ theory of contagious disease has certainly owed much of its success to the fact that it embodies an ontological representation of sickness. After all, a germ can be seen, even if this requires the complicated mediation of a microscope, stains and cultures, while we would never be able to see a miasma or an influence. (p. 40)

The pathogenic model of medicine looks more favorably upon those disorders that have readily observable causes. These are more *real*. As it has been described above, they are more easily viewed in the objectivity—which is tantamount to being *real*. It is the responsibility of medicine and medical scientists to understand these pathogens, their onset, symptoms, and treatments.

LIMITATIONS TO THE PATHOGENIC MODEL

When medicine is synonymous with medical science, medical conditions can only be defined—that is, they can only be real—in their objectivity. While this was helpful for viruses and bacteria (and Canguilhem's "germs"), this hasn't been helpful in understanding lifestyle-related diseases such as cardiac disease, type-II diabetes, chronic illnesses, and a host of psychopathologies.

Cardiac disease refers to any breakdown or abnormality in the autonomic regulation of the cardiovascular system. The heart pumps oxygenated blood through the blood vessels, delivering oxygen and glycogen to cells. With cardiac disease, there is no foreign germ or pathogen that has entered into the system. Instead, normal elements within the system fall out of balance. For example, cholesterol is a substance produced by the liver that is delivered to cells. It allows animal cells to metabolize certain vitamins and minerals. Too much or too little cholesterol leads to problems, and this process can be tied to diet. When the levels get too high, and the cells all have what they need, the excess cholesterol begins to accumulate in the blood vessels. This accumulation can eventually lead to blockages, requiring the heart to pump much harder or more frequently.

Excess cholesterol is just one example of how cardiac disease is a different variety of disease than Parkinson's. Parkinson's disease is an abnormal deterioration of the basal ganglia near the motor cortex in the midbrain. There is no cure to Parkinson's disease until neurologists have learned how to regenerate damaged nervous tissue. There is also no cure to cardiac disease because there is no invading pathogen—the issue is instead one of balance. The *problem* with excess cholesterol is that it increases the likelihood of a cardiac episode. Medication (such as a statin) can be prescribed to *decrease* the amount of cholesterol produced by the liver. This adjusts the nutrition-cardiovascular relationship in a person with high cholesterol. It is a change to their body. This is not an instance of a cure, but one of risk management. The liver is not infected, and neither is the person's lifestyle. But the combination of liver function and the lifestyle of the person has resulted in an increased risk of cardiac disease.

Lifestyles are not so easily objectified the way a virus or bacterium might be. One does not *have* a diseased lifestyle the way they *have* a virus. There is no pathogen to objectify in order to be treated medically. The lifestyle is not a pathogen. As certain lifestyle choices (such as diet and exercise) are understood *in terms of their relationship to certain medical risks*, they become medicalized. When a dietary habit is related to a decrease in risk, it is understood to be health-giving or healthy, but when it contributes to an increase in risk, it is understood to be heath-decreasing or pathological. Within the pathogenic model of medicine, health is a dependent variable.

Going back a few decades, you will find that few things have been demonstrated more completely than the relationship between smoking cessation and a *decreased* risk of cardiac disease. Despite this evidence, the practice of its implementation has been difficult indeed. Everything has been tried to get smokers to break the habit: increasing the cost of cigarettes, printing pictures of cancer or cardiac disease patients on the cigarette packages, making it illegal to smoke indoors, and so on. Smokers continue to smoke. "Cigarette smoking" cannot be cut out of a person the way a tumor can.

Another well-known risk factor for cardiac disease is obesity (and morbid obesity). These classifications of body mass are named specifically for their increase in probability for cardiac disease. In order to decrease body mass, one must expend more calories than one consumes. This typically calls for a substantial transformation to dietary and activity habits. This medical recommendation is directed at one's energy sources. Whichever diet/activity balance had been found throughout one's life, the balance through which they have found sufficient energy to comfortably handle their responsibilities for the day, must be modified. Since body mass reduction requires a decrease in caloric intake relative to activity levels, this means that one must necessarily adapt to a decrease in available glycogen stores (in order to metabolize fat, the less-efficient energy stores). This leaves one feeling lethargic, hungry, and often in a mental fog. Lethargy, hunger, and mental fog upset the daily routine, and the dieter suffers.

"Diet and exercise" is not the same kind of prescription as a daily statin would be. The latter requires but a single new activity in one's daily routine. The former requires a complete transformation of one's customary habits and routines.

As the leading cause of death in the United States, considerable efforts have gone into *treating* the factors that lead to increasing the risk for cardiac disease. Medications, surgeries, recommendations for dietary and activity changes, as well as a host of additional lifestyle changes have been proposed and tested. As a result, more and more of the contemporary lifestyle has been viewed through the eyeglass of "risk management." For example, relationships, occupations, hobbies, diet, social habits, drinking habits, smoking, relaxing, and spirituality are each viewed as possible factors of cardiac disease risk. These dimensions of life have become medicalized.

The population that is *most* at risk for suffering a cardiac episode is those who have already suffered a major cardiac episode. Even with the valuable learning experience of how serious cardiac disease is, there is a strong unwillingness to amend the "at risk" dimensions of their lifestyles. It is not that medical science is unhelpful, but that the lifestyle prescriptions are substantially more difficult for a person to follow. Even though medical science has traced many lifestyle factors to the increase/decrease of likelihood of cardiac disease, this is not so easily translated into medical advice. For example, telling a person that an electrolyte does not count as their daily water intake is often unhelpful in bringing about a behavioral change.

Another problem with the prescription for changes in lifestyles comes from the model of medicine that began to examine them. By looking for a "cause" for problems such as cardiac disease, the dimensions of lifestyle are necessarily targeted as suspected pathogens. There are so-called unhealthy behaviors that are to be avoided. For example, when the consumption of red meat is correlated with an increase in cholesterol production, it is put on the "foods to avoid" list. This ignores the need for cholesterol in metabolizing dietary nutrition. Along with red meat you will find salt, fat, some forms of alcohol, and sugar. Dietary fads develop that cut out entire food groups, like the ketogenic diet that avoids carbohydrates, or diets that call for cutting out all fats and sweets. With each of these examples, the dietary item is viewed as a cause of cardiac disease: a pathogen that must be avoided. In addition to being almost completely unavoidable, fat, salt, and sugar are important parts of any diet. They just tend to get overconsumed. They are not pathogens by themselves; it is the practice of their consumption that has led to increased levels of risk of mortality.

As the pathogenic model began to target more and more of the Western lifestyle—pathologizing certain foods, beverages, hobbies, relationships, work schedules, and sleeping habits—people began to experience certain dimensions of human experience as off-limits. The list of pathologized lifestyle decisions—things you must avoid doing—was getting so long that people began evaluating every action as whether it increased or decreased the likelihood of a lifestyle-related disease. This leads to a lot of "I shouldn't do this or that." In sum, the outlook was supremely negative: "What am I doing that is possibly leading to my premature death?"

SALUTOGENESIS: DE-PATHOLOGIZING LIFESTYLES

Aaron Antonovsky (1923–1994), the Israeli American medical sociologist, didn't find the pathogenic model very helpful when it came to treating lifestyle-related disorders. Indeed, the focus on pathogenesis (finding the root problem or cause of disease/disorder) has led to a series of foods, behaviors, relationships, and work habits that have become taboo. Based on his research, Antonovsky has recommended that the pathogenic viewpoint do an about-face. Instead of asking "how are my actions possibly leading to my premature death," he has recommended that we ask "how are my actions contributing to my health and well-being?" Instead of looking at everything as potentially pathological, why don't we look at it as potentially salutary (i.e., increasing one's longevity and well-being)?

This reversal is built on the basic existential tenet that each of us may be found somewhere along the continuum between life and death. Every person will eventually die, which means that death is always a possibility: we are always moving toward this pole. But we also are not there yet: each of us has at least some measure of life. As long as we have not yet died, each of us is doing *something* right. The pathogenic model has asked: what are the behaviors, diets, habits, and routines that push people toward the death pole? Antonovsky reverses this: what are the behaviors, diets, habits, and routines that push people toward the life pole?

Salutogenesis is a reminder that no behavior or dietary ingredient is necessarily pathogenic all by itself. Just like too much salt and too little salt are both risky decisions, so too is too little or too much fat. When you add salt to your dinner, Antonovsky does not offer shame or scorn with the pathologizing question "how is this shortening your life?" Instead, he asks: "what is this doing to contribute to your life and well-being?"

In salutogenesis, all of the formerly taboo behaviors are looked at within a new light. Even smoking (gasp!). When we examine the population of workers who are most likely to smoke tobacco and drink alcohol excessively, we find medical nursing staff and restaurant employees. Both jobs require that workers put in long hours on their feet, the management of many tasks that must be carried out in an orderly and often scrutinized fashion, and typically come with a variable schedule (so that there can be no adaptation to a regular routine). How might we *understand* smoking within this context? The 2–3-minute smoking breaks might be the only few minutes that a nurse or restaurant worker gets to him or herself during a five-hour block of a 12-hour shift. What happens when these smoke breaks are eliminated cold turkey?

Antonovsky worked with cardiac disease patients and eventually found an important dimension of existence that predicted whether or not a person would become rehabilitated. He called this dimension "Sense of Coherence." Sense of Coherence is a three-fold awareness a person has of their well-being: understandability, manageability, and meaningfulness. With every medical issue, a person must first understand what is wrong and what will be necessary to become rehabilitated. They must be confident in their own ability to do what must be done— that is, they feel adequate to the rehabilitation task. And they must see the entire episode as a meaningful component of their own development as a person—that is, they must integrate the rehabilitative process into their identity.

With salutogenesis, Antonovsky successfully reorients the relationship between lifestyle and risk of disease. Unfortunately, salutogenesis has not *replaced* pathogenesis. It is simply an additional tool in the medical tool belt that some providers may choose to use.

Salutogenesis is a step in the right direction when it comes to a medical understanding of lifestyle-related diseases and disorders. However, it does not give us the existential dimension of healthcare. This is because *health* and *well-being* are not states that can be worked toward—they are not dependent variables. Health and well-being are names for integrated, meaningful lives. Medical interventions—be they pathogenic or saluto-genic—*intervene* on the integrated, meaningful lives persons have developed and to which they have become accustomed. Interventions always *upset* health and well-being; they do this by medically problematizing health and wellness.

References

Canguilhem, G. (1991). *The normal and the pathological* (C. R. Fawcett, Trans.). New York: ZONE Books.

Roser, M. (2018). Child and infant mortality. *Our World in Data.* https://ourworldindata.org/child-mortality

CHAPTER 3

Reality and Medicine

Abstract This chapter is where the audience is introduced to what the blind-spot in medicine has missed: human existence. Bodies are there, but humans exist; humans are being there. Two dimensions of human being—the concrete world of existence and the abstract world of bodies—are carefully introduced and compared. The world of medical science, with its objective observations, manipulation, and control, takes as its object the material or corporeal body (*Körper*). The concrete body is the one that is lived (*Leib*). Humans can be understood through their concrete experience. Efforts to do so are directed at their existence.

Keywords Medical science • phenomenology of the body • Martin Heidegger • Leib • Körper

The being of humans (such as yours and mine) is fundamentally different from the being of objects (such as tables and chairs). When we say that the table and chairs are *on the patio*, then we understand that they are merely *there*—out on the patio. If you were looking for a place to sit and read the newspaper, you could wander out onto the patio and find the table and chairs there. The table and chairs are *just* there. Now if I were to say that *I* am out on the patio, you would never find me merely there; you would always find me *being there*. It would be most peculiar to find me there the same way that you find the table and chairs—as if I were to be standing

© The Author(s) 2019
P. M. Whitehead, *Existential Health Psychology*,
https://doi.org/10.1007/978-3-030-21355-8_3

there motionless. But even in this case, you would find me both standing *and* motionless. You would also not, in comparison, find the chair standing or motionless. Could you even imagine?

Humans are never merely there, they are always *being* where they are. This means that the quality of *there* matters as well. Projects of reading the newspaper or practicing t'ai chi require very different space accommodations. This means that you and I are always occupying our surroundings in a particular way. If a few friends were helping you move furniture into your apartment, and you realized that the coffee table was *in the way* as your friends tried to move the couch, then you would slide it up against the wall so as to get it out of their way. Now the coffee table is *there*, out of the way. It is way-making with respect to the work of your friends who are busy moving the couch. Now if you then realized that you were also in the way as they continued to move the couch, you might press your back up against the wall so as to take up as little space as possible. You are not just there, pressed up against the wall the way that the coffee table is: you are *being* helpful or unhelpful, actively *taking up* as little space as possible.

Humans are always existing in this capacity: they are always living out relationships with their surroundings. Humans do not just behave or react to stimuli in their surroundings but interact meaningfully. Even a short, polite conversation in the elevator is more than a reflexive interaction with the environment or behavioristic stimulus and response. Saying "hello" or "how are you" are attempts at *being* polite, kind, or social. Sometimes these ontological occupations (i.e., ways of being in the world such as newspaper reading or t'ai chi practice) come into conflict with one another. If you are engrossed in a book when an elevator passenger attempts to engage you in conversation, you may not even realize that they had started talking to you. Because you are absorbed in a book, the rest of the world is present to you only insofar as it is useful to your ontological occupation of book reading. The rest of the world remains in the background—the setting within which your occupation of reading may continue. It remains invisible as the background until it becomes sufficiently distracting enough to interrupt your reading—like if the elevator passenger nudges you in a desperate attempt to get your attention. Suddenly the interaction takes the foreground and the book fades into the background, and you have gone from the ontological occupation of reading to one of social interaction.

Objects in our environment are only ever viewed in terms of their usefulness for our ontological occupations.[1] We can understand that the chair on the patio is useful as a place to read in a manner that is different from its usefulness as a weapon during an altercation. A desk is not cluttered until you cannot find what it is you are looking for, or it is no longer a desk to be used for organization and work but instead a desk to be used as an example of how clean and orderly you keep your office when your spouse drops in to say hello.

The body, as we have already seen in Chap. 2, can be viewed in its objectivity—a certain height and weight, a heart that pumps blood, and a nervous system that metabolizes glycogen. It is also always the necessary vehicle through which you carry out your various ontological occupations. It is that through which *being there* becomes possible. Mucous in the sinus cavity traps irritants and allergens in the air you breathe. Like the windshield of your car or the screen on your smartphone which you always use but seldom notice, you ignore your sinus barrier until it becomes a problem. Diseases and injuries always happen *through* this living and active body. They happen *to* bones, muscles, and cells, but they are only ever *experienced* as major or minor transformations to the ontological occupations which have become your routine. A broken metatarsal in your left foot makes normal walking very difficult and painful. The ontological occupation of mobility between office desk and the parking lot is transformed. Instead of walking to my car while I am thinking of what I will be making for dinner, I am now painfully aware of my gait, foot placement, as well as how my awkward walking pattern must look to any students who may happen to look up from their phones to witness me in my condition. However, sitting at my desk and reading e-mails or participating in a conference call remains unaffected. I am able to become fully absorbed in these activities without impediment. The *experience of injury and disease may be understood as illness.* Ontologically signified as pathogens, diseases affect the body; existentially experienced, illnesses affect the person.

It is possible that an injury or disease is objectively present without interfering with a person's ontological occupations. Hypothetically, deterioration of long-distance visual acuity would not be noticed by a person who is never required to make long-distance visual discriminations. In an

---

[1] It has become fashionable among contemporary continental philosophers to imagine the world of objects from the latter's perspective, but even these thought experiments are carried out in service to the project of de-anthropocentrizing philosophy.

actual example, my wife had a patient who had complained of indigestion. Phenomenologically, indigestion restricts one's ability to sleep, exercise, or comfortably engage in effortful activity. During the part of the examination where she palpates the stomach region, my wife felt a large mass on the patient's kidney. An MRI revealed a softball-sized tumor. The tumor represents an important medical condition. Since it did not change the patient's ontological occupations, she did not *experience the tumor as an illness*. It wasn't until the size of it began to press upon the stomach, leading to indigestion, that she began to experience the tumor as a problem so that it could be identified and operated on.

You and I do not *feel* a broken bone or tumor the way it is palpated (or viewed by way of MRI) by a medical provider. When we notice it at all, it is only ever as a change in what we can or cannot do. This is true even if all we wish to do is to sit and enjoy a cup of coffee in the morning. Despite its simplicity, enjoying a cup of coffee is likely impossible with a constant throbbing radiating from the foot or a concern that the coffee will lead to indigestion. Since medical science has been developed around the manipulation and control of the body *in its objectivity*, it is incapable of understanding or treating the patient *in her existentiality*. The latter is a blind-spot. Indeed, medical science has viewed existential reality as *less real* than objective reality.

To summarize from the previous chapter, the reality that matters to a suffering person is not the reality that is privileged by medical science. The reality of medical science is reality in its objectivity—that is, the reality that yields to measurement, manipulation, and control. Medical science cannot, in principle, validate a person's suffering. It can only confirm the presence of a particular injury or pathogen. The reverse is also the case. A person cannot, in principle, *experience* a particular injury or pathogen *in its objectivity*.

Consider the following: if I experience pain in my jaw when I chew breakfast cereal, medical science cannot confirm or deny this. I experience the pain as an inability to bite down as hard as I normally do while I absentmindedly chew my cereal, absorbed in the task of reading e-mails or talking with my wife. Instead of being present to the e-mails or conversation, I am repeatedly brought back to the chewing process, as I now have to make an effort to avoid chewing with a sensitive molar. A physician cannot see this; she can only choose whether or not to take me seriously about my pain and discomfort. This is a social, political, or perhaps ethical action, but not a medical one. Instead, medical science can look for neurophysiological problems or structural abnormalities that could be understood to be responsible for the suffering. For example, there might be an ambiguous dark spot on the root of a molar in the affected jaw, which *might be* a bit of decaying tooth. I cannot *feel* tooth decay any more than I *feel* my cerebral cortex as I judge the speed of oncoming traffic while making a left-hand turn. Tooth decay is state of organic-chemical breakdown of enamel and dentin, which has certain empirical qualities recognizable by a dental specialist. "Pain while chewing cereal but not pita bread" is not one of those qualities. "Tooth decay" is thus a certified dental-medical observation that is outside of my expertise.

In the above example of the patient in whom an MRI revealed a substantial tumor, we can assume that the tumor had been growing there for at least a few months if not years. This means it had been there, receiving oxygen and blood from the cardiovascular system and without any apparent influence in the "patient." She was not, of course, a patient person at this time, because there was no suffering with which she was forced to be patient. Nevertheless, she *had* cancer—a possibly fatal medical condition. The tumor, and by extension her medical condition, is real *in its objectivity*. In her experience the medical condition is not a reality. She is probably surprised at the radiologist's so-called discovery. Furthermore, when the oncologist surgically removes the tumor, the now patient will have a surgery from which she will have to recover, with its associated pains and prescription for rehabilitation. The only suffering she will experience will be a result of the treatment: she will hurt *only once there is no longer anything medically wrong with her*. In this latter case, the stitches that hold together the incision site are objectively real, and therefore the patient's experience of pain at the surgery site is validated medically. But as she learns from her oncologist, she is fortunate to have had the surgery—which she can only trust is true. Once again, this is a social, political, or even ethical action, but not a medical one.

Once more, the reverse can also be the case—as with chronic illnesses such as chronic pain. Before it became "chronic pain," the ambiguous medical category it is today, this had been called "idiopathic pain." Idiopathic refers to a problem for which the objective cause is unknown. The pain, it seems, is only evident to the patient, who in many cases experiences this at debilitating levels. Idiopathic pain cannot, by definition, be validated in its objectivity. There is no identifiable underlying neurological, physiological, or chemical signature by which medical scientists can *objectify* the pain. There is nothing that can be objectively manipulated. It is often apparent from the changes to the patient's life that there is something wrong, but these changes are not as readily discernible as is a tumor on a kidney. In this case, the condition has a robust existential reality, but an invisible objective reality.

The existentially invisible condition (tumor) can be objectively identified and treated with relative ease. Medically, treatment is always directed at a body in its objectivity. This is easy in this case because the problem is easily circumscribed: you might even imagine a dotted line separating the tumor tissue and the healthy kidney tissue. It is obviously complicated when blood vessels are passing between each bit of tissue, but the point here is that the condition is empirically observable. The existentially real condition cannot be validated in this manner, and as such there is nothing to "treat." The obvious rejoinder is that the provider must *treat the person.* Not with a medical intervention, of course, but by trying to understand what it is that the patient needs. As psychiatrist and chronic illness expert Arthur Kleinman (1988) has observed, a practitioner must seek to "understand how a person and the person's world affects and are affected by a disorder" and that "this is the surest way to provide humane and effective care to the chronically ill" (p. 96). Unfortunately, as he points out, this often complicates the disease-focused treatment plan.

Heidegger's (1962) philosophy of human being is of obvious importance to medical practice as well as medical science—provided medical science is willing to amend its axiom that medical reality can only ever be reality in its objectivity. As Boss read Heidegger's description of *Dasein,* he immediately recognized something fundamental to the practice of medicine, but it also seemed to land just outside of his cognitive grasp. He needed some help making the connection clear. Fortunately for Boss, Heidegger was still alive, and did not live terribly far from Zollikon.

Psychiatry

It must have been weird to have a seminar where psychiatrists—trained in the assumptions of modern medical science—received a lecture from a philosopher who explained that the significant dimension of human being would always be just beyond the grasp of their medical model. Many of the question/answer sessions revealed that Heidegger's lectures were accepted only after considerable difficulty and skepticism.

Psychiatry itself has an interesting background in medicine. Dating back to the nineteenth century, psychiatry has been the field devoted to those problems that had found no other classification in medicine. It includes those abnormalities for which no underlying cause can be objectively found. This can be understood as an instance of an *illness*—which is the experience of an impairment to a person's life such that some or many of their ontological occupations have become impaired—but for which there is no identifiable (and thus medically treatable) cause. Take *hysteria*, for example. In 1910, Sigmund Freud presents Breuer's case of Anna, who had exhibited among other symptoms sudden paralysis of the extremities, an inability to drink water, and troubling hallucinations. The medical assumption, Freud explains, was that the origin must certainly be neurophysiological. However, since the precise neurophysiological *pathogen* or abnormality had not been discovered, there was no treatment. That is, until Breuer had observed improvement (and even elimination) of symptoms through the treatment of talking—that is, a so-called talking cure. How talking proved to be an intervention of a presumably neurophysiological impairment was uncertain, but it was also the only acceptable explanation medical scientists could produce.

What happens is that talking seems to be helpful for the treatment of Anna's hysterical symptoms. There is a noticeable change to Anna's normal routines of being able to drink water and express herself, and talking about the trauma of watching her father drift away into a painful death seems to be helpful in returning Anna to her normal, everyday self. *To this explanation, Breuer adds* that he has cured a neurological problem with a new treatment. There is no evidence before or after she is treated that Anna had been suffering from a neurological disorder, but this does not stop Breuer from discussing it this way.

Psychiatric medicine is the category of presumed medical conditions that have not yet been discovered in their objectivity through medical science. *If*, for example, a lesion had been discovered that is associated with hysteria, then the latter would cease to be a psychiatric disorder and would become a neurological one. This is also what will happen if a neurologist ever "discovers" depression. The latter is a present-day psychiatric diagnosis: an illness for which no underlying physiological cause has been associated, but which is also assumed to be neurophysiological in origin. This is what happened with neurosyphilis in the early twentieth century.

The symptoms of neurosyphilis are similar to those of Alzheimer's: changes in motor abilities, personality, dementia, confusion, disorientation, and so forth. By themselves, these symptoms can be understood as an illness for which no disease had yet been discovered. Like hysterics of the same time, these neurosyphilitic patients would undergo considerable behavioral transformations. In 1927, physiologist Julius Wagner-Jauregg discovered the neural infection responsible for the disorder (which is associated with syphilis, the sexually transmitted disease) and treats what then becomes known as neurosyphilis. For this, he wins the Nobel Prize for Medicine. Because its physiological origin had been discovered (after all, psychiatrists had suspected that there was a cause in there somewhere), *it became a neurological disorder and ceased to be a psychiatric disorder*. You would no longer go to a psychiatrist for treatment but would seek the help of a neurologist. Since it is built on the assumption that behavioral problems are *actually* neurophysiological problems, even in the absence of evidence, Thomas Szasz (2008) has called psychiatry "the science of lies."

PSYCHOLOGY AND PSYCHIATRY

The same neurophysiological assumptions that dominated the understanding and treatment of psychiatric disorders had also been occurring within the field of psychology at the beginning and into the middle of the twentieth century (and indeed, even today). Since the late nineteenth century, psychology has been concerned with mental faculties such as thinking, remembering, feeling, and perceiving. As early as 1894, with the publication of Oswald Külpe's *Grundriss der Psychologie*, psychologists committed themselves exclusively to understanding the neurophysiological conditions that were understood to be responsible for mental faculties.

Just as the body of disease (the presence of a pathogen) differs from the body of illness (the way it is experienced), so too does the experience of tactile perception differ from the underlying neurophysiology. When feeling the weight and texture of paper stock that a book page has, you do not *feel* several thousand sub-dermal pressure corpuscles or the neurochemical activation of many thousands of nerve cells. This is the case even though cognitive neuroscientists can map the precise neurophysiological network that makes the sensation of touch possible. What you feel is the fragility of the onionskin-thin pages of a Bible, the brittle and sandy pages of an aging first edition of *Sein und Zeit*, or the smooth and durable pages of a book you have just purchased. If you're absorbed in the book as you read it, you likely do not notice the paper stock at all, as it is irrelevant to what is printed on its pages. In this last case, you are not aware at all of the many thousand sub-dermal pressure corpuscles and so forth, even though they are busy releasing neurotransmitters to other neurons.

When applied to psychology, Heidegger's philosophy encourages a focus that is directed at the manner in which the body (with its many neural and physiological systems) and mental faculties are taken up. This is the reason why Boss sees in medicine and psychology the same existential foundation.

Existential Medicine and Psychiatry

As the Zollikon Seminars were underway, Boss began writing what would become *his* magnum opus: *Existenzgrundlage von Medizin und Psychologie* (1970/1974). The second edition was translated into English as *Existential Foundations of Medicine and Psychology*. As described already in the Introduction of this book, Boss realized that something was absent from the dominant model of medicine at that time: and it is "precisely the essence of the way people behave among themselves in their daily lives"— that is to say, it is humans in their being.

In *Existential Foundations*, Boss goes into considerable depth regarding the case of a former patient of his, Regula Zürcher. Zürcher's case reads very much like the hysterical patients that Freud described in his Lectures on Psychoanalysis. For over a decade and into her late 20s, Zürcher suffers from eczema, constipation, menstrual problems, and a general physical weakness. Every conceivable specialist is called upon to review her case and to treat whatever condition she might *have*. Boss explains,

> The patient kept losing weight until she had dwindled to eighty-three and one-half pounds (she was five feet ten inches tall). The small army of six doctors treating her was prepared for the worst. The internist she trusted most told her pointblank that he was at his wits' end. (1979, p. 5)

Upon physical examination, there was no evidence of disorder or abnormality through which the attending physicians could make meaningful sense of the severity of her symptoms. It was not *in* her body. They certainly played out through her body—that is, many of the symptoms could not manifest but through her body—but they could not be understood as pathophysiological. With nothing to lose, Zürcher seeks out a psychotherapist. What emerges from her conversations with her psychotherapist is a history that had not been understood by the team of medical doctors who were treating her. It was a story that is familiar to those who have suffered from chronic illnesses such as the neurasthenics and pain patients described by Arthur Kleinman (1988). Zürcher's life had been disordered—hers was a joyless and oppressed one. The youthful vitality, love, and intellectual curiosity that were being stifled by her numerous so-called medical conditions had also been stifled by the strict formality of her parents.

With his book, Boss argues for a new starting point for medicine and other studies which share human being as their subject matter (such as sociology or psychology). The popularity of its first edition among physicians and human scientists alike shows that his insights were well received by a broad variety of disciplines.

To found medicine as an existential practice means to begin with existentiality as the nature of humankind. Boss explains,

> We declare that only man *exists*. This is not to say that material, inorganic nature and nonhuman beings—animals and plants—are in any sense unreal, insubstantial, or illusory because they do not so *exist*. We merely state that the reality of these nonhuman realms differs from that of human existence, whose primary characteristic is *Da-sein* (literally "being-the-there"). (p. xxix)

What Boss describes is the difference between existential reality and objective reality. It is not that medical science with its emphasis on objectivity is incorrect or unhelpful, but that it is blind to the "being-the-there" of the human. While it did not seem important to consider this human dimension in the nineteenth-century practice of medicine, many chronic cases came to demand it.

Freud had recognized the importance of nonobjective dimensions of patients' realities—such as their past experiences, their expression of desire, and the meaning of their actions. He began integrating these into his treatment plans—unraveling the patient's knotted mind, he believed (i.e., *psychoanalysis*). Freud and his followers understood that these conversations were serious medical procedures and required extensive training and practice in medical science in order to carry them out. Even today, the practice of psychoanalysis without a medical doctorate is called "lay psychoanalysis." While the diagnosis *and* treatment deals entirely with existential reality, it is understood that the procedures are indicative of an underlying pathophysiology. That is to say, there is an assumption that the foundation of existential reality is necessarily objective reality. The causal connection is an assumption of medical science. As it has been described already, objective and existential realities cannot be translated one to the other.

Boss suggests that we stop making the metaphysical leap from existential problem to pathophysiological problem. This is only revolutionary because medical science (and Western society more broadly) has privileged reality in its objectivity. *Real* has come to be defined only as that which has empirical extension in space and time. Like Freud many decades earlier, Boss observes that some problems occur to a person's way of being (existence) and these cannot be evaluated in their objectivity. Moreover, they can be treated at the level of being (or existence) by talking about existential meaning. The difference between Boss and Freud is that Freud *believed* that what he was doing was consistent with medical science. After all, psychoanalysis (like psychiatry, clinical psychology, and other mental health professions) deals with diagnoses, best practices, and probabilities of cure. Boss does not think it necessary to attribute the conversations he has with patients to medical science but allows them to remain on the level of existentiality.

By allowing the conversation about psychopathology to remain on the level of existentiality reality, it frees up the medical researcher to understand *how* a particular illness is lived. Instead of focusing only on what the possible physiological conditions might be for a particular disorder, researchers can begin to understand the breadth of existential impact. They can look not into the feature of disease, but those of illness. That is to say: they can look not at how the body has been affected by disease but may look at how a person's life has been affected by illness.

As mentioned above, this is particularly important for those illnesses that are understood *only in their existential reality*—such as chronic illnesses. The case could also be made for the long list of mental disorders that are defined by the *Diagnostic and Statistical Manual of Mental Disorders, 5th Edition* (*DSM-V*; American Psychiatric Association 2013). The *DSM-V* defines disorders in their subjectivity—specifically as changes to the patient's way of being (i.e., the existential dimension of human being). As long as they are listed in the *DSM-V*, they are currently diagnosed only in their existentiality. However, the majority of recommended treatments play out on the level of the body in its objectivity (such as through changes to the patient's neurochemistry). Like neurosyphilis described above, as soon as these disorders are understood and diagnosed pathophysiologically, they will cease to be mental disorders and become neurological or physiological disorders.

An Adequately Human Conception of Medicine

The more strictly our description of the traits of healthy existence adheres to their human character, the more solid this existential foundation for medicine will be. ... It is a consideration of everything about the actual mode of human existence that has as far been overlooked by, or been inaccessible to, the natural sciences. (1979, p. 85)

The conception of medicine which privileges diseases, injuries, and disorders in their empirically objective reality is adequately biomechanical in nature. It privileges humans in their objectivity. As described above, objective reality cannot be experienced directly: it is not translatable to human existence. The latter is where illnesses reside—the experiences of suffering and of the breakdown of one's day-to-day routine. Considering medical problems in their existential reality would begin with the meaningful world of the patient's experience: this would be an adequately human conception of medicine.

In every disease or injury, there is a change to the world of the afflicted person. That is to say, in even the most objectifiable medical disorders, such as pneumonia or Huntington's Disease, there is a person whose life has been transformed. An adequately human treatment takes this transformation into consideration. This is not said in order to justify the reclassification of diseases in their objectivity as illnesses of life, but to recognize that diseases are also experienced—something that is essential to understand for rehabilitation purposes.

Unfortunately, the privileging of the objectifiability of medical disorders has been maintained even when a medical disorder has not yet been understood to have empirically objective properties. "What caused it" has become more important than "how must this affliction be *lived*?" Telling a recently paralyzed man that his spinal cord has been severed and that this has eliminated all efferent, afferent, motor, and somatosensory information flow from his lower extremities misses the mark of addressing the significance of the substantial life change that awaits him and his family.

The causal description of illnesses has been practiced even in the absence of objective evidence. Depression is described and treated as if it were a neurological or neurochemical disorder despite substantial disagreement about what, exactly, has *caused* it. This is to say nothing of the diagnosis, which asks how a depressed person's existence has changed. With tens of thousands diagnosed with this existential change in the United States alone, it would seem as though it is worth exploring in its existentiality. Instead, it is assumed that the most important thing that can be said about it is what has caused it. Boss explains the counterintuitive nature of this with the following:

> Anyone who insists on taking a genetic approach [i.e., indicating the preceding cause] without having first sufficiently explained the nature of the phenomenon under investigation is ignorant of the very thing whose origins he is looking for, like someone trying to reach a goal he has never glimpsed. (p. 195)

An adequately human conception of medicine would not attempt to begin with medical conditions in their objectivity or as a sequence of cause and effect. Instead, it would begin with an understanding of the nature of human being and how this nature can become a problem for a person. It begins with research into what it means to be human and how this humanity is lived by a particular individual. An adequately human understanding of a medical disorder can only begin by first understanding the pre-disease or pre-injury existence of the individual, and how this has been transformed in illness. An adequately human methodology for healthcare is presented in Chap. 7.

REFERENCES

American Psychiatric Association. (2013). *Diagnostic and statistical manual of mental disorders* (5th ed.). Washington, DC: APA.

Boss, M. (1979). *Existential foundations of medicine and psychology* (S. Conway & A. Cleaves, Trans.). New York: Jason Aronson.

Heidegger, M. (2008). *Being and time* (J. Macquarrie & E. Robinson, Trans.). New York: Harper Perennial. (Original translation published in 1962).

Kleinman, A. (1988). *Illness narratives: Suffering, healing, and the human condition*. New York: Basic Books.

Szasz, T. (2008). *Psychiatry: The science of lies*. Syracuse: Syracuse University Press.

CHAPTER 4

Existence and Health

Abstract This chapter introduces the concepts of health and well-being. These concepts can only be understood existentially, and they are absurd when defined objectively. This chapter draws on the work of American physician and philosopher of medicine, Drew Leder, who explains that when healthy, the lived body is absent from experience. There is no concrete experience of health. Health is merely the ability to become absorbed in one's routine. This is called "well-being" by German hermeneutic philosopher Hans Georg Gadamer. Like Leder, Gadamer argues that health is not any special category, but the ability to carry on with one's routines without being hindered.

Keywords Gadamer • Leder • Existentialism • Illness • Health • Well-being

Health is difficult to define because it can only be understood in a person for whom the concept of health is irrelevant. The activities in which a healthy person engages are manifold, and are specifically uninhibited by bodily injury or disease. It would not, of course, occur to such a person to think about themselves as healthy. Health, as late German philosopher Hans Georg Gadamer (1996) has observed, is merely well-being. And "what is well-being if it is not precisely this condition of not noticing, of being unhindered, of being ready for and open to everything?" (p. 73).

© The Author(s) 2019
P. M. Whitehead, *Existential Health Psychology*,
https://doi.org/10.1007/978-3-030-21355-8_4

American physician and philosopher of medicine, Drew Leder (1990), describes this view of health in his aptly titled book *Absent Body*. In it he explains just how difficult it is for patients to communicate when and how their health has become a problem for them. He argues how experientially, health is the absence of any problem. When it becomes a problem, it does not announce itself in a particular manner such as "cardiac weakness." Instead, one experiences that one's energy levels are low, it seems difficult to get a satisfyingly deep breath, one's appetite is unreliable, and so forth. One does not encounter a disease in the way it would be understood by a medical scientist, but as problematic transformation of his or her day-to-day routine.

This is not how health is treated by modern medical science. To the latter, health is a value or good that can be increased or decreased, bought or sold, as well as measured and tested in a laboratory. To medical science, health is empirical and quantifiable. On the one hand, the experimental treatment of health benefits from the reliability and validity of the scientific method. On the other hand, however, the experimental treatment of health begins by negating its subject matter—namely, health-as-well-being. That is to say, all of the benefits of experimentation are lost when applied to health, because health cannot be measured.

In the pathogenic model of medical science, health is the absence of pathogen or disease. Health is understood as that which militantly combats disease. But nowhere in the "de-pathogenic treatment" is health considered. Indeed, with a blood-born pathogen, a diagnosis is made only once the phlebotomist has witnessed through a microscope the pathogen in a drop of the patient's blood. What the expert finds is the presence of a given pathogen. Treatment is directed only at this pathogen. If the medical scientists were genuinely interested in health, the discussion would begin only once the patient person began to experience a disturbance to her daily routine. Only at that moment would her health begin to present as a problem for her. Of the many possibilities that occur to the patient for what might be responsible for her disturbance, a variety of medical issues might be among them. Based on the description of the disturbance, the physician would rule out possible medical problems, which only then may lead to a consultation from the phlebotomy specialist.

In this rendering of the health-conscious physician, the practice of medicine is understood to be a person-centered art and not an impersonal science. Gadamer explains how the modern natural sciences are built on the capacity to produce effects. The influence and importance of such practices are proportional to the effects produced. This production is how the value of medical practice is conferred. By contrast, the art of medicine emphasizes balance and equilibrium—qualities possessed by the patient and not the physician. The physician is the guide for these processes to come about. "[W]hen the act works," writes Gadamer, "suddenly everything seems to happen spontaneously, lightly, and effortlessly" (p. 37).

The artful practice of medicine does not revolve around the medical scientist and her expert manipulations, but the processes of equilibrium which belong to the patient. As such, it is the health of the patient that is under consideration, not the health as defined by medical science and which, by extension, can only be obtained through expert medical practice. Otherwise, patients become committed to the idea that health is a product that can only be given by a small handful of experts. Such patients become dependent on their physicians for the provision of care. For Gadamer, such an instance must be viewed as a failure of medicine. "[Providers] must know when to stand back. For they must neither make the patients wholly depend on them, nor needlessly prescribe dietary or other conditions of lifestyle which would only hinder patients from returning to their own equilibrium of life" (p. 43).

Health is restored only once the patient returns (or, perhaps better still, adapts) to a routine of life such that her health fades into the background, allowing her projects of being a mother, wife, and/or coworker to occupy her attention. Or as Gadamer puts it, "Genuine success is accomplished in medical practice at just that point where the intervention is ultimately rendered superfluous and dispensable" (p. 37).

With this in mind, it is evident that it is the patient herself who is the subject of health, and not her blood. "Doctors must be able to look beyond the 'case' they are treating and have regard for the human being as a whole in that person's particular life situation" (p. 43). An illness, disease, or problem can only ever be understood by first understanding the person whose way of being has become disturbed.

MEDICAL BODY, LIVED BODY

In English, there is a single word for the organic-physical substance of which the human being is comprised: body. There is no distinction between your living body that is currently absorbed in the activity of reading and the stiff body beneath the examining spotlight in the coroner's office. These are, of course, very different meanings of the word body: one is living and the other, lifeless. In German, there is a separate word for each. The living body is *Leib*, and the lifeless body is *Körper*.

When understood as *Leib* (life; *leben*: living), the body is alive, active, and engaged. It is the body of experience (*Erlebnis*); it is the body I identify as myself. It is the sensing, feeling, and interacting body. It is not simply the body that has a pulse or in which organic activity unfolds, but also the body through which a person has meaningful engagements in the world. It is the body through which one sets out to mow the lawn and the body that rests in satisfaction afterwards. It is the body that aches with hunger and loneliness. When an over-excited puppy delivers a skin-breaking bite during play, it is through this body that one cries out: "you bit *me!*"

When understood as *Körper* (corporeal), the body is inert, inactive, and lifeless. This is the body as a physical object: the body that takes up space. With the dimensions of height, weight, volume, density, hardness, and so forth, it is the body of modern science and the body of medical science. Medically, the corporeal body with a beating heart is alive. The living quality is not personal, but biomedical. When the heart beats too quickly, it is tachycardic and never "excited." When it beats too slowly, it is brady-cardic, and never "lethargic."

With *Leib* and *Körper*, there are always two ways in which I can experience my body. I can view, massage, and manipulate my right leg as a muscular-skeletal limb, and I can do the same with your leg (*Körper*). But only through my leg do I have an experience of being viewed, massaged, and manipulated (*Leib*).

As a concept of medical science, health is concerned with the body as a corporeal object. The medical evaluation of "neurocognitive disorder" assumes that a lasting impairment to a neurocognitive apparatus has taken place, or that the latter has somehow become damaged. The recommended medical course of treatment is directed at this neurocognitive impairment. The medical body can only ever be understood in terms of its corporeality: empirical, measurable, and quantifiable.

Existentially, health is experienced as well-being. This is not to be understood as a particularly good feeling when compared to the day-to-day average, but as no distinct feeling at all. Well-being is not an evaluation the way that a neurocognitive impairment is. Well-being is simply the ability to continue as I have been, engaged in the projects that matter to me and that characterize my life. In doing so, I never encounter my leg directly as a muscular-skeletal limb. Insofar as I am healthy, my leg disappears into the projects of ambling about while lecturing in the classroom, jogging along a wooded trail, or driving to the supermarket. The lived body can only ever be understood in terms of the lived world of the person, through his or her *experience* of space, time, embodiment, other persons, and one's attunement or mood. These five modes comprise the existential structure of the lived world.

Existential Modes of Being

Modern science has been built on the procedure of observing the physical properties of things by breaking them down into their smallest parts. By first understanding the smallest parts of a given object, these may be added together to understand the larger object itself. These part objects can be observed in relation to one another and until all of the different objects in the universe have been scrutinized. However, as soon as you begin to break the existence of human beings down in this fashion, you immediately lose the very existential quality you were after. Existential structure is not chemical or neurological. It cannot be a brain state because it is not experienced this way. There is nothing to look "at" that will yield the existential structure of human being. It is something that must be dealt "with."

To explain experience by way of brain states, nervous system activity, or neurotransmitter chemicals is to confuse human experience with the conditions for experience. The brain does not *remember*, for example. Composed of nervous tissue and blood vessels, the brain metabolizes glycogen and cycles neurotransmitters. *Remembering* is a process of relating to past experiences and making present once more what was for a time absent. You and I relate to our past by way of remembering. We understand our experiences on the background of these memories. Meanwhile, the brain metabolizes glycogen. Without this metabolization, we could not relate to our past in this manner. It is a necessary condition. But metabolization is not itself the relationship between past and present. The relationship is a dimension of the existential structure of human being.

The existential structure of human being is always already with you and I. It informs me as I write and informs you as you read. It is in the thread of continuity of experience, and it supplies the framework of meaning within which our experiences unfold. Scientific procedures are unhelpful for making this structure clear. This is problematic because critical thinking in education is often oriented around the scientific way of looking at the world. For example, Isaac Newton is famous for describing the modern scientific world-view: that the universe is like a box with the three dimensions of extension (space) and the one dimension of duration (time). Everything that is, is within these dimensions. Moreover, it is assumed that these dimensions have the qualities of homogeneity and repeatability. Real objects have extension in space: length, width, and height. They take up a finite amount of space and last for a finite amount of time.

Modern science has been working within these presupposed dimensions of space for nearly four centuries. Time has been mostly ignored, as quantum physicist Lee Smolin has observed in his 2014 book *Time Reborn*. Modern science, particularly as applied in medicine, has only recently taken up the dimension of sociality: like how the presence of a network of social support expedites recovery in cardiac disease patients (Allan and Fisher 2011), even though cardiac health was previously understood to be an exclusively physiological domain.

Humans may be understood within these dimensions as well, but the experience of space and time are something altogether different. Once we can begin to see the difference between objective space and time as scientific dimensions on the one hand, and human spatiality and temporality as existential dimensions on the other, we will begin to see the presence of a few more dimensions as well: sociality, embodiment, and mood.

Spatiality In modern physics, space is a starting assumption. Space is the arena necessary for an event to unfold. The physical measure of mass is literally the amount of space an object takes up. Physical objects take up space. Human bodies may also be understood as having such and such a mass or taking up so much space. However, thus rendered, a living body is no different from a lifeless one, such as a cadaver in a biology laboratory.

A human being does not just take up space, but also occupies space. To human beings, space can only ever be understood as the arena of a particular activity. Insofar as it is encountered at all, space is encountered as "space to...." As an object, a physicist will observe that my desk takes up a considerable amount of room in my office. But to me, my desk is not a space-taker but a space-giver: it supplies a level surface at a height comfortable for me to sit and write and answer e-mails. Through it I am able to more comfortably and conveniently carry out my identity as college professor.

We do not relate to ourselves, our world, or to one another as objects on a plane of x and y dimensions. We are not spaced apart by units. Space is not itself an absence of stuff, but an opportunity to be inhabited by movement or our projects of being. To human beings, space can only ever be lived space. A classroom cannot be defined by its entryway and adjacent windows: that would be a description of a watchroom: a room whose purpose is to be occupied by those who look out the window. A classroom is a space for the meeting between students and instructor, and must be set up in a manner that facilitates this. The *space* of the classroom is defined by the way in which it comfortably accommodates students, their need to see the teacher, and to take notes, the way it accommodates the teacher, her need to see her students, and a means of illustrating the examples she gives during the lecture. The projector screen, blackboard, and rows of desks would each *take up space* in a dance hall, but in the classroom, they *make space*.

Space can also only ever be encountered *in time*. The kitchen is not 18 meters away, but a ten second walk from where I am seated on the couch. This distance grows when I am tired or when I have an injured leg. The distance to campus is not 20 kilometers, but about 20 minutes without traffic and 35 when there is construction on the highway beside my house; it is a 90-minute run.

Temporality Experiences always unfold *in time*. That is to say, time is also lived. The duration of time that we experience is not the time that is measured by a stopwatch or clock. Not all minutes are lived equally: some minutes fly by like seconds while others seem to stretch on for an eternity. Minutes are never long enough to a person who wishes to accomplish a great deal all at once. Minutes are too long when a person is waiting around for something better to happen.

Experientially, time can never be wasted—it can only ever be spent with persons or things. A five-kilometer jog with my dogs may take 24 minutes in duration when measured by a stopwatch, but this is not how I experience it. The 24 minutes is a mode of being-with-my-dogs-along-the-country-road. If I have not made sufficient time for my dogs, then I may be rushing, or focusing on what I would rather be doing. In such a case, I might be physically with my dogs, but my attention, focus, and interest lie elsewhere (such as with a book I am reading or a chapter I am writing).

Finally, an important temporal dimension that shapes the meaning of our lives is that our time is always finite: we will not live forever. If there was no limit to the moments we could experience, then there would be no push to prepare for or start a job, to make friends, or to start a family—these tasks could be drawn out infinitely into the future and would therefore lose any sense of urgency. The perceived need to *do all things at once* is anxiety—a phenomenon that has a temporal dimension (Aho 2018). Depression, too, may be understood through its temporal dimension—perceived as a slowing of time-to-be-something in particular (Aho 2008).

Embodiment In modern scientific disciplines that concern the human— such as medicine and, more recently, psychology—it has been customary to assume a division between that which has extension and that which does not. It is assumed that there is a body on one side and a mind on the other. Such a division presents a conundrum for anybody who wishes to understand the human subject. Wundt (1896) and Whitehead (1920) are two exemplary philosopher scientists who tried to resolve this problematic assumption.

Existentially, however, we do not begin with an assumed division between mind and body. Instead, it is recognized that the body and mind are always already together. In the previous example of running with my dogs, it could be argued that my mind and body were separated: my body was jogging alongside them while my mind was back in the office working through a problem. Were you to see me, however, you would notice, only by looking, that I am not attentive to or affectively present with my dogs. You would gather this by observing my bodily engagement with my environment. Indeed you may even ask "where did you go just now?" My attentive absence would be given to you through my bodily engagement (or lack thereof).

The access I have to the world is only granted through the body that I am. I do not *have* a body—I *am* a body. Feelings of loneliness and enthusiasm unfold as embodied experiences, not as clouds of thought that emanate from my pineal gland. Sight, smell, taste, touch, and hearing are points of phenomenal access I have to the world, and I can only understand the latter through these points of contact. The world does not cause my experience of it; my experience is a manner of bodily engagement with the world of things. We cannot understand vision as a consequence of eyeballs. This is to assume that the eyeball and its supporting neurological network cause our vision. The eye does not see; a person sees. Eyeballs are complicated organs of photosensitivity. Seeing is a human way of interacting with the world. Without the eyes, we still feel and hear our way throughout our surroundings—seeing, as it were, with our hands and ears. Touch, taste, hearing, and smell are also human ways of interacting with the world. Organs do not accomplish these actions—humans do.

Sociality We are social beings. We exist in relation to others. Our sense of personal individuality is a product of this primordial awareness of and relationship to others.

The words of this book are not for an internet thing or a generic course on qualitative research methods, but for a handful of scholars and students whom I imagine wish to engage the human subject matter in a manner that appreciates existential depth. It may seem like the words are meaningful in and of themselves, and that their generation is a purely cognitive event, but this is not how conversation works. When responding to a question, we do not construct our response by putting together semantically related words into grammatically accurate and logically coherent phrases. If that were the case, then we could always reproduce a conversation identical to one we have just had. But this is unlikely except for the case of a routine conversation where little is meaningfully shared. Conversation is a social interaction. We are not merely producing words in response to other words but interacting with another person. We recall not the specific words we have said the way that a recording device would, but what it was we tried to express. As such, the social context is a necessary factor of speech.

Sociality is not only limited to speech but encompasses our entire being-in-the-world. That is to say, being is always a with-being (or being with). Philosopher Emmanuel Levinas famously demonstrated this in his book *Totality and Infinity* where he explains how through the very process of childbirth, a being's existence is always already a social one.

Mood We also live in an affective (i.e., an emotionally charged) relationship with the world. This quality transforms what we notice and, by extension, how we engage the world. If I am having a lousy day, I cannot help but notice the lousiness in all that I behold. The food that I eat is not life-giving sustenance, but a thrice-daily chore and drain on my checkbook. The soreness in my knee is an excuse to skip my afternoon run and complain about my boredom.

These perceptions change when I am having a good day: meals are not daily chores or checkbook drains, but opportunities to create something together with my wife. My knee is no longer a cause of my self-pity, but a reminder to back off a bit during my workouts or to stretch my legs out more regularly. Because our awareness of the world of experience is always mooded in such a way, this is also commonly referred to as attunement.

We often imagine that we are upset because the things of our world have made us this way. I am angry and frustrated because something happened on my drive this morning that angered and frustrated me. In this manner, I am nothing more than an effect brought about by an environment of causes: I thus play no role in the meaning my life has for me. Existentially, we realize that it is precisely the opposite: I am angered and frustrated during my drive, and because of this, I perceive the driving events that occur as angering and frustrating. For example, if I am already running late, then everything that happens *makes me run late*. This doesn't happen if I am running five minutes early.

EXISTENTIAL DIMENSION OF ALL MEDICAL INTERVENTIONS

For every injury, disease, or virus, there is a transformation of the above dimensions of existence. For example, in suffering from a torn hamstring, one does not deal with a mere leg injury. The torn muscle limits one's peculiar manner of being-in-the-world. Walking up a flight of stairs, standing up from a seated position, and moving about throughout the day suddenly appear as challenges that must be overcome. The now-injured person is usually blind to these as behaviors as they generally dissolve into other activities such as "going to the bathroom" or "walking to the office." Now they must "go to the bathroom with a stiff, painful gait." The injury upsets the habitual processes that define one's lifestyle. Furthermore, we do not need x-ray verification to see these changes take place.

The injury is not limited to the damaged tissue but extends to the entire life of the person. As Gadamer (1996) would say, one's well-being is damaged. Therefore, in order to understand the impact of an injury, we cannot look only at the tissue damage, but must look at the complete transformation of the personality that has taken place (Goldstein 2000).

Imagine that I am a trained concert pianist and have just been in a terrible automobile accident that has resulted in nerve damage in my hands. After a long and complicated surgery, I have regained full motor control of my hands. Unfortunately, now my hands are numb of sensory feedback. I can move them, but I can no longer feel the keys. I cannot feel the piano as I play it. The medical problem is resolved and I am given a clean bill of health. Moreover, neurologists cannot see my numbness, but can only take my word for it. Aside from the numbness, everything can return to normal. The speed and accuracy of my fine motor control is restored to normal, and, because she is a thoughtful, patient-centered provider, the doctor has even brought in an upright piano to my recovery room to demonstrate that I can still control the dynamics of the keys I'm playing. But I cannot feel the piano anymore.

Miraculously, the medical problem has been resolved. What remains is a personal, private problem. It is something that medicine cannot touch, and it surrounds the structure of meaning my life has for me and my potential for activity within it.

A recommended surgery that makes it difficult to type quickly will be harder to accept for someone who takes pride in their writing; a treatment that has a side effect of lethargy will be harder to accept for someone who cares for young children. The examples that I am leading with are undeniably existential, but they are intended to set up many common issues that have previously been difficult to understand.[1]

My wife runs a clinic in the rural southeast. The single most prevalent medical problem she encounters is obesity. Patient histories always begin with "obesity," and a host of medically related problems such as high blood pressure, type-II diabetes, varicose veins, high cholesterol, and various other circulation problems. The medical recommendation always involves a change in diet. The recommended changes are always affordable, simple, and easy to follow. In many cases, a nutritionist is available for additional consultation. In three years, there are only a handful of cases where patients have followed the medical advice and made dietary changes. It is remarkable how quickly these patients are able to be off of their blood pressure and diabetes medications when they follow such recommendations.

The prevalence of obesity is not unique to the rural southeast. The United States leads the world in body mass index, with the combined percentage of overweight and obese adults climbing higher than 71% (National Institute of Diabetes and Digestive and Kidney Diseases). Obesity numbers are growing in American children as well. Life expectancy has also begun to decline.

---

[1] It is here that Boss emphasizes that *any* medical problem is always a problem of one's relatedness to the world. Pain is not an organic problem, but a change in one's ability to relate to one's world in a familiar and meaningful way.

The difficulty of adapting to a dietary change is understandable to any-body who has tried to go on a diet. After a few days of enthusiasm and excitement, things eventually have a way of returning to what was normal before the diet began. That is to say, lifestyle change is not easy because it requires a change of who you are. This is where a medical recommenda-tion is insufficient, and why Goldstein observes an existential dimension present in every treatment (even a routine medical procedure).

When faced with a new developmental crisis, a person has two choices. The first choice is to commit to the lifestyle that has worked out thus far—it is predictable, safe, and familiar, but it is also limited. Because it limits growth and self-actualization, the first choice is existentially pathological (this is also how Goldstein has defined "pathology"—anything that is lim-iting to organismic growth). The second choice is unpredictable, possibly unsafe, and unfamiliar, but it has the benefit of growth. Either choice is understandable: who can be ridiculed for wanting things to remain as they are when, by and large, this seems to have worked out? A parent or clini-cian cannot coerce another person to grow; it must be their decision, because *they* are the ones with everything to lose.

Existential therapists deal with problems of life: they consult with per-sons who are trying to more fully inhabit their lives. Doctors deal with physiological problems: they consult on issues that are medical. But all medical issues have existential dimensions because they always include a change in the structure of meaning a client has for his or her life.

If Samantha has an accident that leaves her paralyzed, then she must relearn how to live as a paraplegic. It is common to think of this medical problem as follows: "Samantha + paralysis." The assumption with this is that everything remains the same except for the parts of her body that have changed. In this conventional medical conception, the paralysis bit is the bit of pathology that must be corrected. "Samantha" is still in there, and she will be found shortly, at least as soon as this new problem has been worked out.

This medical conception of the paralysis problem ignores the eminently important existential dimensions: Samantha must relearn who she is by integrating this new condition into her identity. For a while she will have to encounter the world as "Samantha + paralysis"—a detail she will be reminded of while getting dressed, navigating her kitchen, and passing people in the street. Each of these is a learning experience that can contribute to identity growth, provided she integrates them. In the beginning, it may be difficult to make coffee in the morning, because the ingredients are now in hard-to-reach places. During that moment, Samantha's paralysis becomes a problem for her. She experiences her paralysis as limiting. But eventually she will learn how to solve this problem—through a new technique of reaching, use of grabby instrument, or a reconfiguration of her kitchen. With each adaptation, she learns, changes, and grows. Eventually, such problems will slowly disappear. Each of these problems will be difficult, but with each lived solution, she will slowly begin to integrate her paralysis into her identity. Eventually, she will once again be "Samantha," but qualitatively different from pre-injury Samantha. She will become a new person (like the boy who has discovered his masculinity for the first time). Just like pre-injury Samantha, she will know her strengths and limitations (some of which will have changed). She will also continue to experience moments where her life becomes a problem for her, just like pre-injury Samantha. They won't be problems because of paralysis, but problems of her life, because she no longer differentiates between the two. She will have transformed her identity. She will still have meaningful relationships (which may also have changed), and she will still find meaning and purpose in her life. This is Goldstein's concept of "self-actualization," familiar in circles of humanistic psychology.

If, however, she has tried to remain "pre-injury Samantha," then she will never grow. She will always be a person for whom paralysis is a problem. As you can imagine, rehabilitation can go two very different ways. Medicine cannot heal this problem anymore than it can heal the lifestyle problems that are contributing to a decrease in life expectancy. If the patient does not understand her situation and does not wish to grow through it, there is very little that medicine can do to help her. With billions of dollars being spent on treatment plans and patient compliance programs, there is precious little attention paid to the meaning of the patient's incipient life change.

References

Aho, K. (2008). Rethinking the psychopathology of depression: Existentialism, Buddhism, and the aims of philosophical counseling. *Philosophical Practice, 3*(1), 207–218.

Aho, K. (2018). Temporal experience in anxiety: Embodiment, selfhood, and the collapse of meaning. *Phenomenology and the Cognitive Sciences.* https://doi.org/10.1007/s11097-018-9559-x.

Allan, R., & Fisher, J. (2011). *Heart and mind: The practice of cardiac psychology*. Washington: APA Press.

Gadamer, H. (1996). *The enigma of health: The art of healing in a scientific age* (J. Gaiger & N. Walker, Trans.). Stanford: Stanford University Press.

Goldstein, K. (2000). *The organism*. New York: Zone. (Original work published in 1934).

Leder, D. (1990). *Absent body*. Chicago: University of Chicago Press.

Whitehead, A.N. (1920). *The concept of nature: The Tarner lectures delivered to Trinity College*. CreateSpace Publishing.

Wundt, W. (1896). *Gundriss der psychologie*. Leipzig: Wilhelm Engelmann.

CHAPTER 5

Medicalization

Abstract This chapter describes what happens when the existential concept of health is objectified. The term for this is medicalization. In short, medicalization reverses the medicine and well-being relationship: Instead of understanding that medicine is in service to well-being, well-being is now in service to medicine. As such, preventative medicine asks individuals without any impairment to make changes that affect their well-being. One's routines are inhibited for the sake of not having their routines inhibited. Instead of seeing health as the absence of medical treatment, it has become synonymous with medical treatment. This includes pharmaceutical regimens as well as so-called healthy lifestyle choices. A dissident of modern medicine, Ivan Illich, is used to describe the gravity of these consequences.

Keywords Medicalization • Iatrogenesis • Ivan Illich

As we have seen already, the existential dimension of human being is not as tidy as the objective dimension. Existentiality cannot be neatly summarized or publicly verified the way that objectivity can. For example, the personality and lifestyle changes by which clinical depression is diagnosed by the *DSM-V* (APA 2013) are achieved only through subjective assessment—first through their description by the patient, and second through the attending clinician who either does or does not believe the patient's account. A great leap is made when the attending clinician categorizes the unique transformation of the patient as depression. The many possible nuances of change that the patient has observed in herself are reduced to one psychiatric development. To categorize the patient's experience in this manner is an instance of abstraction: to generalize something that is by its nature singular. The alternative would be to make a unique clinical observation for every patient who presents with symptoms that include anhedonia and working each as a separate case with separate recommendations. Given the many-thousand insurance codes that already exist for medical treatments, this is an unlikely direction for psychiatry to turn.

The use of abstractions is helpful in the practice of medicine—it allows providers to use a single category for the many-thousand possible combinations of the symptoms of depression. But there are a few problems that follow this practice. It implies, for example, that depression may be treated homogeneously—despite its many possible combinations of symptoms. The problem that I will spend the rest of the chapter discussing is what happens when the abstraction begins to *hide* the unique characteristics of the singular case in question. This problem has been called, variously, "vicious abstractionism" by the American philosopher William James, the "fallacy of misplaced concreteness" by the English philosopher Alfred North Whitehead, "abstractification" by the American sociologist and psychoanalyst Erich Fromm, and "hypostatization" by the German philosopher and phenomenologist Edmund Husserl.

The experience of chronic lower-back pain is not localized to the small of one's back but extends into the suffering person's life. Consequently, a father who can no longer hold his daughter will have a very different experience of this pain than the brick mason who cannot work as quickly or for as long as he once could. To homogenize these lifestyle transformations as "chronic lower-back pain" misses their unique impact on each person and thereby *obscures the helpful course of rehabilitation* (or intervention, if necessary). Moreover, it is assumed that each man *has* some physiological, neural, or orthopedic problem that is in principle localizable and measurable, even though chronic pain is defined by the absence of any objective problem. Each person suffers in a way unique to him or herself, and this uniqueness is camouflaged by the generalized medical category. That which is lost through this process of abstraction are the qualities of concreteness: the chronic lower-back pain *as it is experienced* by each man. One cannot lift his daughter and hold her close, and is thereby impotent in his role of father-as-protector. The other cannot exhibit his work-ethic—that upon which his reputation has been based. Instead of viewing the existential transformations in their concreteness, these two unique events are homogenized based on allegedly the objective characteristic they share: pain in the lower back. The *localizability* of pain replaces the concrete meaning in the event of suffering. William James (1909) has called this "vicious abstractionism." He writes,

> We conceive a concrete situation by singling out some salient or important feature in it, and classing it under that; then, instead of adding to its previous characters all the positive consequences which the new way of conceiving it may bring, we proceed to use our concept privatively; reducing the originally rich phenomenon to the naked suggestions of that name abstractly taken, treating it as a case of 'nothing but' that concept, and acting as if all the other characters from out of which the concept is abstracted were expunged. (Chapter 13, Paragraph 7)

Vicious abstractionism can occur in any domain, provided the concrete dimensions of personal experience are lost in their reduction to some category based on a single, "salient or important feature." When the salient feature is an objectified medical category, this process is called medicalization.

MEDICALIZATION

As soon as a given disorder or disease has been investigated by medical scientists and its defining qualities discovered or corroborated, it becomes an artifact of medicine. The discovery or corroboration comes with a state-licensed stamp of medical approval. When you are suffering with difficulty breathing, trouble sleeping, and a terrible cough, you do not yet have a medical condition. If you were to see a physician, s/he would first have to check for mononucleosis, pneumonia, upper respiratory infection, or another possibly fatal condition. As an official medical procedure, the tests can only be conducted by a person with a state-given license to do so. For example, my artist neighbor could listen to my wheezing and diagnose me with mononucleosis, but this would not allow me to conclude that I have the medical condition of the same name. Were he to pretend to be a licensed physician and diagnose me as such, he would be arrested as a medical fraud—a quack—and my condition would remain undiagnosed. The test is a way of identifying whether or not the *objective characteristics* of the medical condition are present. The symptoms that you experience are irrelevant; the diagnosis is only made once the test reveals a particular medical condition *in its objectivity*. The objective attributes that are measured are the salient features of the disorder. That I cannot complete a full sentence or comfortably walk up a flight of stairs are not salient except for directing the medical scientist toward the most likely cause.

This medical procedure is helpful for identifying and treating medical conditions. Its helpfulness is particularly apparent when dealing with pathogens—offending viruses, infections, and bacteria. It has become so helpful with treating these, in fact, that it has become increasingly uncommon to die from such pathogens, as we saw in Chap. 2. The control of viruses and bacteria is an impressive credential that belongs to modern medicine.

The success of the pathogenic model has made it seem like the perfect solution to all medical conundrums. One must only identify the invading pathogen in its objectivity and engineer treatments to specifically target it. Unfortunately, as I have explained, this is not very helpful when it comes to lifestyle-related diseases—the kinds that are the leading causes of death today.

Modern medicine specializes in diseases. Diseases are the results of a pathogen such as a virus or a structural abnormality in the living organism such as a tear in the tissue of the heart. Modern medicine operates by localizing the problem within the system and resolving the issue (thereby curing the disease). This is most noticeable in diseases such as pneumonia, which was, at one time, the leading cause of death in the Western world, until antibiotics such as Penicillin were found to be effective in its treatment.

Medical interventions were once required only when diseases were present. A runny nose or a week of lethargy was understood to be within the range of normal human experience, but bouts of coughing with an elevated body temperature required treatment. In the last 70 years, treatments have become a way of life. Now so-called treatments are routinely prescribed in the absence of any medical condition. It is in this way that medicalization has insinuated itself into our personal lives.

The change in the nature of medical treatment is due, partly, to the way in which the nature of diseases has changed since the beginning of the twentieth century. It is no longer common to die of a pathogen or infectious disease. Modern medicine has done a wonderful job eradicating these once leading causes of death. Despite this success, after centuries of its steady incline, the life expectancy has actually begun to go down. The diseases that currently stymie medical providers and scientists are *lifestyle-related diseases*. Lifestyle-related diseases do not work the way that pathogen-based diseases do. Pathogens can be isolated and treated by a physician, lifestyles cannot.

Lifestyle-related diseases include those that stem from the decisions we make about what we eat, how active we are, our relationships, how we spend our time, and the quality of the life we maintain. Cardiac disease, the leading reported[1] cause of death, is not the result of a miniscule cardiac pathogen. It is the result of many years of eating a poor diet that is high in sodium and saturated fats, prolonged sedentary periods of inactivity, and a general state of heightened physiological arousal in those for whom rest is the exception, not the rule (i.e., sympathetic nervous system activity or stress). Patients who have suffered a major cardiac episode (such as a heart attack) are told that they must make changes to their lifestyle. Taking a daily statin (to reduce cholesterol produced by the liver) is itself a change in lifestyle, however minor. It is an addition of an activity into the daily routine. But medical advice in cardiac disease patients extends well beyond this. Prescriptions are given for healthy and supportive relationships, healthy activities such as walking through a meadow or practicing yoga, healthy foods such as leafy greens and raw vegetables, and healthy expectations for oneself while at work or home. Such prescriptions are based on decades of medical research which have demonstrated the positive relationship they share with so-called healthfulness.

These are not instances of medicine becoming more existential, but of bits of the existential dimension being slowly kidnapped by medicine. The concrete and meaningful experiences that unfold in a person's life are being sorted into abstract, medicalized categories. As this process happens, more and more of our lives are experienced as medicalized. Consequently, our lives become less and less unique and personally nuanced; they become less concrete.

You and I do not need to have suffered a heart attack in order to experience our lives as medicalized. Eating an apple-a-day has left me feeling proud of myself since I was ten. It is not an apple-to-satisfy-hunger, but an

---

[1] It is necessary to add the disclaimer "reported" because cardiac disease is often listed when the cause of death of a person under medical care is uncertain. It is much easier to report that a patient has died due to cardiac complications when they had actually died during surgery, even if that surgery was on their kidneys or liver.

apple-to-combat-illness (even if I feel perfectly fine). I might even imagine the waxy surface of the apple skin cleaning the plaque from my teeth as I bite into it. This, of course, is not something I can experience in its concreteness. I feel the apple's crunchiness in its resistance to be crushed between my teeth. I taste its sour and sweet flavors, and feel its juices splash around in my mouth. I do not feel the vitamins being metabolized any more than I feel my individual cells being hydrated. My experience of eating an apple has been replaced by the medicalized health concept "apple-eating."

Actions such as apple-eating begin to tell me less and less about myself, just as the behaviors of others begin to tell me less and less about them. The consumption of food tells little about cultural practices and social fellowship, and more of self-medication through the regular manipulation and structure surrounding dietary fads. Salt is used in moderation in order to prolong life, and prolonging life is the implicit goal of medicine (regardless of what may be said about quality of life or the desire to live forever).

Other medicalized bits of life include an afternoon walk which contributes to one's daily step total, a ten-second pause to relax while at work, and a compassionate response to a loved one. Each contributes its part in the ongoing battle against disease. Wine is consumed for its antioxidants, kale for its nutrient density, and light beer is understood to be easier on the liver and kidneys than heavy beer. A dog is a social-anxiety-reducing companion and gardens are there to dissipate stress. More and more dimensions of life are seen through the glass of medicalization. Through it we are taught to be ever vigilant against stress, the boogeyman of holistic medicine.

As they become increasingly medicalized, our lives begin to look less and less familiar to us. They become less and less personal. Instead of actions reflecting our unique character and personality, they reflect the generic and medicalized character and personality of "health." We have categories of health and un-health, ease and dis-ease, and we become well practiced at placing more and more of our experiences into these categories.

Instead of resulting in decreases in the consumption of goods and services from the medical industry, more people than ever are actively receiving treatment for potential risks. Treatment always comes with a transformation of the person. *When this transformation is in service to medical health, a bit of the person becomes medicalized. This happens bit by bit until my relationships to my wife and dogs have become methods of self-medication.*

I want to remind you that there is an important part of this "health-life, ease-disease" conversation that has been left out. It is a part about which you and I are aware: it is the expression of meaning and purpose in human being. It is the quality of existence. This goes untouched by medicine. It will never and can never be operationalized or medicalized.

To the familiar list of biomedical fixes in service to health that alienate a person from her existence, I will add the newer list of health-psychological fixes to character and personality that are increasingly also understood to be in service to health. I will remind those of you who see this transition (from biomedicine to biomedical health psychology) as a blessing that introducing the personal into medicine does not *humanize* medicine; it *medicalizes* humanity. *Programs* are engineered to de-stress one's work life, *practices* are tested for increasing empathy and compassion in relationships, and *techniques* are provided to alter faulty thinking tendencies. When these are discussed within the context of medical health and wellness, they become alienating to the person to whom they are in service. They separate from the person all that is personal. When did it become the case that quality relationships are in service to a longer, healthier life? Quality relationships are the *reason to* live, not *in order to* live.

ILLICH'S "MEDICALIZATION OF LIFE"

There are many works from which to choose that concern the medicalization of everyday life, including the collection of the same name written by late psychiatrist Thomas Szasz. Szasz chose the title "medicalization of everyday life" with Freud's famous book, *The Psychopathology of Everyday Life*, in mind. In his book, Freud lets his readers in on a haunting secret: that they slip into brief and minor fits of psychopathology every day. Freud transforms normal waking behavior into evidence of imminent psychosis, declaring how we must always worry that psychosis lies just around the corner. Szasz explains that the title of Freud's book could just as easily have been titled *The Everyday Normalness of Psychopathology*. But this, he admits, wouldn't have been nearly as sinister.

The problem of medicalization echoes the scare of psychosis that Freud accomplishes. But in medicalization, it is disease and suffering that awaits us all, not psychosis. Instead of the everyday normalness of suffering—that is, the notion that suffering is often a normal part of life, it becomes a medical life sentence for which one should spare no expense to avoid. If one is at risk of potential suffering, then one must seek immediate treatment. English psychiatrist David Healy (2012) explains that patients are increasingly being treated for medical risks with the same kind of urgency in current medical conditions. By increasing the medical salience of risk *factors*, the number of potential patients increases exponentially. There is always some probability that a certain condition may await a given person. Treatment of potential medical issues has become a way of life. Indeed, failure to seek treatment for risk factors is likely to be vilified—an act akin to suicidal ideation. Patients must sign a consent form if they turn down a recommended course of treatment. It is along this line of thinking that medical critic Ivan Illich writes his seething manifesto *Medical Nemesis: The Expropriation of Health*.

In the preface to the 1995 edition of *Medical Nemesis*, Illich explains that his original aim in 1975 was to show how "the fundamental pathogen today is the pursuit of health as this has come to be culturally defined in late-industrial society" (p. v). In reflection upon this goal he writes, "I did not understand that in the age of systems management, this pathogenic pursuit of health would become universally imposed" (pp. v–vi). For Illich, the process of medicalization and healthcare has become pathogenic in itself. Rather than *discover* and treat diseases and injuries, it has invented conditions for which treatment becomes necessary.

Illich organizes his relentless criticism of modern medicine around various forms of iatrogenesis. Iatrogeneses are instances wherein medicine, which is in service to life, contributes to life's decay. If a patient dies as a result of a medical procedure, then the death is an iatrogenic one. For example, if during a routine root canal, a patient develops a bacterial infection because an instrument was not properly sanitized ahead of time, then the infection is an iatrogenic one. To organize this work around iatrogeneses is to let his audience know that Illich will be holding no punches. It is his way of reminding his audience that institutionalized medicine and healthcare are the problems.

His criticisms of modern medicine are summarized neatly by the following quote, "The fact that modern medicine has become very effective in the treatment of specific symptoms does not mean that it has become more beneficial for the health of the patient" (pp. 80–81). Similar to the position of Gadamer (1996), who explains that the body will always come to equilibrium and health on its own, Illich maintains that the best that an attending provider can do "is to convince his patient that he can live with his impairment" (p. 80). The goal of modern medicine, as Illich sees it, is to turn healthcare into a commodity for consumption. In order to do so, they must first convince the public that health and wellness are goods to be purchased, and second that they are crucial. If a patient suffers from a heart attack, an emergency room physician can save the patient's life; so too can a physician surgically remove a bowel obstruction from an infant thereby saving the infant's life. Like a trip to see a psychiatrist or the solicitation of a tree-trimming service, life-saving medical interventions are goods to be purchased.

Illich finds that medicine has taken this commodity value of medical interventions too far. If a patient's LDL cholesterol level is elevated, then this may indicate a certain probability of suffering a cardiac episode. However, when an attending physician explains to her patient that the patient must begin taking medication in order to lower the LDL cholesterol levels, something else is happening. The physician in this situation occupies a role beyond that of medical specialist. She begins to occupy a role that is more suited to a pastor or guardian—one who counsels others on matters of morality and what is good. That which is medically solvent has become increasingly conflated with moral justness and righteousness. Following medical advice is what one *should* or *ought* to do.

By succeeding in this, Illich finds that modern medicine has betrayed the Hippocratic oath, and not without consequence. Medicine is by far the most widely consumed good in the United States, and the medical providers (and their office staff) are among the highest paid—attracting scads of capable students every year. Illich summarizes many of the absurd growths in medical spending. Even though they were initially described four and a half decades ago, they are still most impressive.

Since 1950, the cost of keeping a patient for one day in a community hospital in the United States has risen by 500%. The bill for patient care in the major university hospitals has risen even faster, tripling in eight years. Administrative costs have exploded, multiplying since 1964 by a factor of seven; laboratory costs have risen by a factor of five, medical salaries only by a factor of two. The construction of hospitals now costs in excess of $85,000 per bed, of which two-thirds buys mechanical equipment that will be made obsolete in ten years (pp. 50–51).

The medical industry rakes in gobs of money while an increasing percentage of people in industrialized (or medicalized) countries become consumers of healthcare. This means that they make adjustments to their lifestyle *in service to their health*. It is precisely within this detail that the irony of health-as-commodity is evident: conceived this way, healthcare accomplishes the opposite of health. Recall in Chap. 4 how health was defined simply as "well-being," or the state where the concept of health is the furthest thing from one's mind. When changes are made to one's life *in service to* health, then health is exchanged for a commodity. In this case, it is the promise that one will be better off undergoing a change in lifestyle or routine. The promise "being better off" is the commodity of health-care, and it accomplishes the opposite of health, because the latter becomes the focal point of one's activities. Instead of dissolving into the back-ground, "health" occupies the foreground.

If a healthcare intervention were to succeed, one could not have any direct experience of it. There is no concrete experiential value of health, since health is precisely the quality of unnoticeability. It is not surprising that interventions which exact a noticeable change are perceived to be more helpful than ones that actually restore one's well-being—wherein one has forgotten that there was ever anything wrong to begin with. If a pharmaceutical (or even cognitive-behavioral) regimen results in a positive experience, then it seems to have done something rather than nothing. Ironically, the positive "something" that has resulted is conflated with health or wellness (the benefits of healthcare), and a patient becomes reliant on the system for help in the future.

Finally, it would not be fair to blame all of this on the medical providers themselves. At least in the United States, pharmaceutical companies are busy advertising various illnesses and risk potentials to the lay public through the television, magazine subscriptions, and on digital media. By the time they arrive in the medical examining room, they have already been sold a certain bill of goods: namely, that health is an achievement that might lie right around their next corner.

References

American Psychiatric Association. (2013). *Diagnostic and statistical manual of mental disorders* (5th ed.). Washington, DC: APA.

Gadamer, H. (1996). *The enigma of health: The art of healing in a scientific age* (J. Gaiger & N. Walker, Trans.). Stanford: Stanford University Press.

Healy, D. (2012). *Pharmageddon*. Los Angeles: University of California Press.

James, W. (1909). *The meaning of truth*. New York: Dover Publications.

CHAPTER 6

Existential Health Psychology

Abstract This chapter describes where this conversation fits within the history of psychology. An existentialist rendering of health and well-being fits into the functionalist school of psychology and may be seen in William James as well as many of the humanistic psychotherapists. Existential health psychology is introduced as a new healthcare occupation akin to hospital chaplains, but without any religious presuppositions. Their job is to complement the existing medical professionals. While medical science is directed at the body, existential health psychologists will be directed at the person who must overcome new medical issues, and to help patients adapt to their new, post-injury personalities.

Keywords Health psychology • Existential psychology • Existential psychotherapy • Rehabilitation studies

Like modern medical science, psychology has been focused on human being in the latter's objectivity and to the neglect of existentiality. But this was not only the case. To understand this, we have to reexamine the earliest proposals for psychology as it was just getting started.

About 130 years ago, William James of Cambridge and Wilhelm Wundt of Leipsig were introducing research for a new discipline in the academy: psychology. Taking the root words *psyche* and *logos*, the new discipline would study the spirit of human being. James and Wundt each proposed

© The Author(s) 2019
P. M. Whitehead, *Existential Health Psychology*,
https://doi.org/10.1007/978-3-030-21355-8_6

projects of sufficient breadth, examining both body and mind. James called these the conditions necessary for experience (i.e., the body) and the psychological faculties themselves (i.e., the mind). Wundt used the terms "objects of experience" (body, stimuli) and the "experiencing subject" (mind). Each proposal included an experimental science of the body as well as an introspective component, which attempted to empirically observe mental processes. By the close of the nineteenth century, however, psychologists had dedicated themselves to the experimental practice alone. This meant that the processes of thinking, perceiving, remembering, and so forth were ignored *in the degree that they were meaningful to the person* and *in the degree to which they were lived*. In an attempt to counter this trend and identify what was missing, James wrote an article titled "The World of Pure Experience" where he proposes "radical empiricism," a method aimed at the breadth of human psychology—even that which cannot be adequately operationalized and made into in/dependent variables. Radical empiricism failed to catch on.

After four to five decades of interpreting psychology as the experimental science of body and behavior, a new group of psychologists wondered at the possibility of a psychology of meaning and purpose—that is, an adequately human psychology. The prefix "human" was only necessary due to the habit of removing everything that had resembled *human being* from the study and practice of psychology.

Humanistic psychology was a reaction against what psychology had become during its first 60 years. By the 1950s, more than a half a century of psychologists had expertly atomized, mechanized, and scientized every empirical manifestation of human being. Whatever may have been left was discarded, most famously in John Watson's (1913) "Psychology as a Behaviorist Views it." The courageous breadth of projects outlined by William James and Wilhelm Wundt never materialized, and psychology became an appendage of the natural sciences while psychiatry became an appendage of the medical sciences.

Humanistic psychology emerges at a time when it had become inconceivable to *humanize* the human subject matter. Humanistic psychologists congregated around the position that humans are not mere mechanical assemblages. Humans are not *mere* carbon chains and neurological impulses; they are not *mere* objects of experimental study. They are, of course, carbon chains and neurological impulses, but adding these objective properties together does not give us the breadth of human being. Something is left out of human being when the latter is reduced in these manners. Psychological clinicians, scholars, and students had grown dissatisfied by the manner with which the discipline of psychology had abandoned its subject matter, and they began to speak up about it. Charles Bugental summarizes this shift in an article published in 1962 in the *American Psychologist*, calling it "A New Breakthrough." The resistance came from individuals who had decided to take the psychological subject matter seriously once again, and to countenance fully an area of life that modern science had not only ignored, but one that it was incapable of taking seriously: human existence.

Like medical science, the natural sciences have been organized around a single defining principle: the systematic examination of that which is publicly observable. We can find an appropriate exemplar in physics: physicists publicly examine the physical world—the active and interactive world of objects that have mass, density, boiling point, volume, and so on. The physical properties of objects are publicly verifiable, belonging, it seems, to the objects themselves.

There are many areas of study dedicated to the world in its publicity. Some scientists study insects while others study the world of freshwater or saltwater fish. However, despite the many areas of systematic public examination, there are still areas of human experience that are left untouched. These include those experiences that do not give themselves over to public observation—ones that are private. For example, if you were to be slid backwards into an fMRI machine as you are reading this book, cognitive neuroscientists could demonstrate publicly the exact combination of neurocognitive apparatuses that are being employed, while various other instruments could be used to indicate your level of physiological arousal. The sum total of your reading behavior could be analyzed and evaluated by teams of psychologists, each with their own unique area of expertise. No matter how many psychologists evaluate you at this moment, there is something that will always be left out of their analyses: the ten or so sets of eyes examining your precise neurophysiology and behavior will not yield your experience of reading right now, and the boredom or curiosity it incites.

Perhaps in the event of book reading this private detail is irrelevant, but there are many important areas in which this detail is exceedingly relevant, as in the contemporary practice of medicine. In 1934,[1] Kurt Goldstein tried to explain the importance of this private, personal, and existential

---

[1] The German was translated into English in 1964.

detail present in every medical treatment. Goldstein explains that a patient must always understand that she is choosing between a limit of freedom or a decrease in suffering. That is to say, a patient may either accept full freedom of expression—what Goldstein calls an increased milieu—and continue suffering, or they may accept a reduction of both freedom and suffering. As such, the patient must always be in charge of her treatment. Abraham Maslow has applied this wisdom fruitfully in motivational theory; Rollo May has applied this wisdom fruitfully in emotional theory; now we must apply it fruitfully in the practice of patient care—an area of practice for which psychologists are uniquely suited. It is essential that psychologists recognize the areas that require their specialty, because there are fewer and fewer of these to be found.

In the decades following the humanistic revolution in the 1950s and 1960s, the practices of science began to change. The change, of course, predates the articles written by Maslow, Rogers, and other figures in humanistic psychology, and it has also occurred in physics, biology, sociology, zoology, and so on. If "mechanism" is the term that usefully describes the projects of modern science, then we can call the mid-twentieth-century transformation "holism.[2]" Holism maintains that it is not always the most helpful solution to understand the smallest parts of a system first, but that sometimes you have to view the entire system as a whole and in its context with other systems in order to understand it. Humanistic psychologists have observed the "whole person"; sociologists observed the social behavior in its socio-cultural-economic-political milieu; physicists began observing the subject-object interrelationships; and medical providers began observing health as a complicated interrelationship between dozens of factors that include, but are not limited to, biology and chemistry.

Looking back, it seems as if the humanistic psychologists have gotten their way: no longer is it customary to view part processes *to the exclusion* of situational and contextual factors. There are outliers of course, such as the *DSM-V*, but any remaining calls for a 1950s–1960s-style psychological revolution are no longer necessary (Whitehead 2017).

The holistic revolution adds something to the philosophy of mechanism. This is an improvement, but the private quality of human experience is still being left out. To include the latter, a second humanistic revolution is in order—an existential-humanistic revolution. This chapter looks at how this might be accomplished within the field of health psychology.

---

[2] This is a distinction borrowed from Gendlin and Johnson (2004) and Gendlin (2009).

To be sure, there are health psychologists, psychiatrists, medical social workers, and therapists at every hospital and in many clinics, but what they are more suited for is medical science. What health psychologists offer are treatments that have demonstrable and publicly observable effectiveness in decreasing mortality, abating disease, or improving measures of health and well-being. Health psychologists address the patient in her objectivity. Existential health psychologists address the patient in her existentiality.

There are two main arguments that I wish to make regarding existential health psychology at this time. The first is broad and concerns the subject matter of psychology. More and more of the realm of human experience have been overtaken by medicine. This is the problem of medicalization described in Chap. 5. The second is carving out a new area of research and practice called existential health psychology. This is not to be confused with an appendage of medicine, but an introduction to a new field concerned with examining an important part of experience that has been historically left out of the healthcare conversation.

EXISTENTIAL ASPECTS OF LIFE, HEALTH

As it has been described in Chap. 2, the objective physical dimensions of an object validate its reality. In medicine, however, reality becomes less well defined. A cadaver has the same kind of reality that a living patient has: both take up space. The possibility of transitioning from living patient to cadaver has certain consequences, and for these consequences, hospitals often employ priests, pastors, and religious figures who are available for consultation. It would be misleading to understand that the priests and pastors are playing a medical role, as these professions land outside the expertise of any medical specialty.

In hospitals, the structure of people's lives either *have already* changed, or are about to change substantially, and medicine is not in a position to deal with or handle this. This is the spiritual side of health, and it requires experts of this type of spiritual study—those who examine the meaningful structure of private experience. This dimension of life change is inherently existential-psychological. It is the crisis known as human development as described by Erik Erikson (1994). It is the construction of new meaning after the reliable structure of meaning, around which a life has been built, has fallen apart or has been upset in some way. This change will not be found in the patient's neurochemistry, their cells and tissue, or platelet count. It also will not be found in the evidence-based operationalization of various life practices such as relationships, thinking strategies, and stress relievers. It is the personal reconciliation of their continued existence within a transformation to their identity. It is a tragic developmental crisis. It is existentialism at the hospital, and consultants are needed.

Existential health psychologists do not need to *replace* chaplains any more than they should replace physicians. Medical providers (and other state-appointed healthcare workers) are there to treat the biopsychosocial health of a patient. When the problems are physiological in nature, they require the expertise of physiologists. For pathogenic medical problems, this will suffice. Additional consultation is needed only when the pathogenic condition becomes a problem for the patient. If I tear my plantar fascia and cannot walk, I will need a podiatrist and possibly a surgeon. These are medical problems that require medical intervention. Such a problem will only require the kind of existential consultant I describe if my medical condition becomes a problem for me. For example, with my torn fascia I may have trouble adjusting my expectations about what I can do around the house and become disappointed with my helpless state. This is not a medical problem, but a problem of living.

Many patients need no additional consultation adapting to a life changed by physical handicap or new pharmaceutical regimen. They follow doctor's orders. Others will. Of those persons who subscribe to a particular religious sect, they will find the support necessary to rebuild a meaningful identity with their religious leader or hospital-appointed chaplain. I am also not recommending that existential health psychologists replace chaplains. However, more Americans than ever identify as "spiritual but not religious." These people are defined by their agnosticism or atheism along with a belief that there is something meaningful beyond themselves. They are skeptical of a religious narrative for constructing meaning around their life change (Cox and Jones 2017). These patients will need help reconciling their existence with the former expectations of their pre-injury self.

Adapting to a Life Change

Existential health psychologists work with medical patients. Otherwise, we would simply be talking about existential counseling. The primary area of practice for the existential health psychologist would be in consulting with a patient as she adapts to a substantial life change. This change can be one brought about through a traumatic incident (such as an accident that has left her paralyzed), or a change that is the recommended course of treatment (such as a substantial change in diet).

The urgency of this issue became clear to me last Fall when I spoke at The American Congress of Rehabilitation Medicine. At the conference, I found that providers earnestly wanted to know how to better understand their patient's decision-making process when it concerns medical advice. Why, for example, will a Type-II diabetic refuse to change her eating habits when doing so will prevent her from losing her toes? Why will a stroke patient refuse to complete rehabilitation exercises when doing so will restore lost motor function? Why is it that a cardiac disease patient will stop taking her medicine when doing so will prevent another heart attack?

What the providers don't realize, at least not yet, is that the such questions are not medical ones. The life they have been trained to preserve is not the personal life of meaning and importance. The answers will not be discovered the way that Penicillin was discovered. These questions are existential. They have to do with the meaning that life has, and the uncertainty, skepticism, and fear that surrounds them. Fortunately, the process of personality change throughout the lifespan is a familiar one to developmental psychologists, and we may look to the latter for guidance on how to best help patients who suffer from medically related incipient life change.

TRANSFORMATIONS OF SELF: EXISTENTIAL-DEVELOPMENTAL GROWTH

Transformation to the personality is not exclusive to post-injury rehabilitation, but it occurs regularly throughout the lifespan. The development of muscular and perceptual coordination transforms a young child's way of being aware and interacting with the world. Imagination and problem solving present first as obstacles and next as openings into greater agency and participation. Shifts in priorities in adulthood transform the background upon which life experiences are meaningfully understood. In short, development throughout the lifespan presents a series of transformations to the personality structure, a process that can be understood as existential growth.

From an existential-developmental perspective, the lifespan may be understood as a series of social, physiological, and cognitive changes to which one must continuously adapt one's personality. Adaptation of one's personality here is synonymous with existential growth. For the most part, the transformations are consistent across persons. French psychologist

Jean Piaget has described four cognitive tasks of children; Erikson has described eight social tasks throughout the lifespan; American psychologist Daniel Levinson describes three primary transitions in adulthood; and so on. In each transition, something has changed for the person such that remaining as the person they were is no longer possible, beneficial, or salutary. The person has two choices: they may resist the transformation and remain existentially stunted or stuck, refusing to actualize their new potentialities; or they may accept the transformation and grow into the new potentialities. Late American existential psychiatrist Thomas Szasz (2010) captures this quality of human being with the following quote:

> Modern man seems to be faced with a choice between two basic alternatives. On the one hand, he may elect to despair over the lost usefulness or the rapid deterioration of games painfully learned. Skills acquired by diligent effort may prove to be inadequate for the task at hand almost as soon as one is ready to apply them. Many people cannot tolerate repeated disappointments of this kind. In desperation, they long for the security of stability—even if stability can be purchased only at the cost of personal enslavement. The other alternative is to rise to the challenge of the unceasing need to learn and relearn, and to try to meet this challenge successfully. (pp. 264–265)

For Szasz, each life stage has its own set of rules which yield its own pearls of wisdom. But aside from their sequentiality, one game never prepares you for the one that follows. One must ever yield to the rules of the new game and allow growth to occur in a new way.

Rehabilitation to an injury or life-altering trauma must be viewed in the same manner. Instead of human development dictating the direction of growth, for the injured person it is the injury and/or trauma that dictates the direction of personal growth. The process, however, requires the same act of yielding in the face of personal inadequacy, and then learning/relearning what is necessary to meet the challenge successfully.

The field of medicine understands this need and has developed a new and decidedly humanistic solution: patient-centered medical care (Morse 2016). Providers have realized that patients need to participate in their treatment, just like Carl Rogers realized that they needed to participate in their own therapy. There are dozens of books, articles, research institutes, and entire conferences devoted to patient-centered medicine, but I maintain that medicine cannot solve this problem. Meaning cannot be medicalized. Patients do not need more solutions. They are drowning in solutions. They need other people who can help them recover meaning in their own lives. Erik Erikson's (1994) eight stages of psychosocial development provide a model of how one can adapt to a developmental life change. They are also useful for understanding the structure of a medically related life change.

In each of Erikson's stages, one must reconcile a change in one's existence with the personal identity to which one had grown accustomed. For example, in the second stage of development, "Autonomy versus Shame and Doubt," a child's mastery of somatosensory experience and motor control becomes problematized by the new development of a willful desire to become a responsible agent. It is no longer enough to merely feel, move, stand, and assimilate the sense environment; now a child wishes to participate in a distinctly personal way and see the impact this makes. The child learns that her actions impact those around her just as others' actions impact her.

By describing these stages as crises, Erikson hopes to demonstrate that there are no solutions to them. This is very important. You do not battle or defeat a crisis. A crisis is only resolved through a transformation of your personality. It is resolved through personal growth. The toddler does not defeat the Autonomy stage by proving that she is in control of all things. Can you imagine? She tries to, of course, which is why the stage is of crisis proportions. Otherwise it would be just another learning experience. She realizes that there are some things of which she is capable, and upon which she reflects with great pride. But there are some things of which she is incapable, and she finds these disappointing. Through these understandings, she grows and becomes more well balanced. In each stage, a new balance must be found, and sometimes it is necessary to make changes to previously balanced tensions.

Existentially, we can understand Erikson's stages as follows: with each stage, a person's life becomes a problem for them in a new way. Furthermore, their life becomes a problem for them in a way in which it was not previously possible. In the stage Erikson calls "Generativity versus Despair," the significance of one's personal identity is decentered. Events no longer revolve around a personal and self-invested interest, but around others, be they children, nieces and nephews, or the next generation. This is not an ego-motivated decision such as "I should be more considerate of my children." The world itself seems different. The way in which weekend plans are considered has changed—viewed no longer only through their significance to you, but how they are understood to impact these newer, younger, others. Consequently, one undergoes an existential shift in meaning, importance, and purpose. The entire personality shifts, ever so slightly, to match this new motivation. As Erikson has observed: for many people, these shifts in perspective typically do not occur without problem.

In short, our lives are already spent adapting to substantial changes. As soon as we find a balance in one area of our lives such as settling into a new job, something changes and a new balance must be found. We might receive a promotion for good work, and then learn that we must now work different hours or develop a new skill set in order to deal with the new responsibilities and expectations. With these changes, a new way of being must be developed; growth must occur.

On this point, it is helpful to remember how Kurt Goldstein (1934/2000) has defined the medical terms "normal" and "pathological." Normal refers to anything that contributes to an organism's self-actualization, and pathological is anything that inhibits this. Failure to adapt to a developmental change (or injury-related change in potential) can be understood as pathological in nature. An example can be found in the toddler who does not get her way and sacrifices her own needs if that means that she can also reject the needs of her oppressor. Less extreme versions can be seen in the type-II diabetic who continues to drink 32 ounces of Gatorade a day as her "water intake" and the stroke patient who refuses to participate in rehabilitation exercises. The change in lifestyle proves too great a sacrifice for extended life. The "cure for life" is not worth sacrificing the current mode of living.

In existential development, the new life balance that is found must be a personal one. It must be discovered by the person who will have to live with it. It is his or her life. A solution cannot come without consulting the patient person: it must be the client's wish. A clinician cannot *make* a patient's suffering meaningful. Meaning cannot be imposed on another person. The patient must create this themselves.

REFERENCES

Cox, D., & Jones, R. P. (2017, November). *Searching for spirituality in the U.S.: A new look at spiritual but not religious.* Public Religion Research Institute. https://www.prri.org/research/religiosity-and-spirituality-in-america/. Accessed 20 Mar 2018.

Erikson, E. (1994). *Identity and the life-cycle.* New York: Norton.

Gendlin, E. (2009). What first and third person processes really are. *Journal of Consciousness Studies, 16*, 33–62.

Gendlin, E., & Johnson, D. H. (2004). *Proposal for an international group for a first-person science.* New York: The Focusing Institute.

Goldstein, K. (2000). *The organism.* New York: Zone. (Original work published in 1934).

Morse, J. (2016). *Qualitative health research: Creating a new discipline.* London: Routledge.

Szasz, T. (2010). *The myth of mental illness: Foundations of a theory of personal conduct.* New York: Harper Perennial.

Watson, J. (1913). Psychology as a behaviorist views it. *Psychological Review, 20*, 158–177.

Whitehead, P. (2017). Goldstein's self-actualization: A biosemiotic view. *The Humanistic Psychologist, 45*(1), 71–83.

CHAPTER 7

Adequately Human: Methods for Health Science

Abstract This chapter describes a methodology for studying healthcare that is adequately human. Building off of the description of health given in Chap. 5, a method is explained that is directed at concrete experience of well-being and deficits to this. Two examples of this are shared: narrative medicine and existential phenomenology. Narrative medicine focuses on the stories that we tell about our lives and our experiences. Illness interferes with how we see our life moving forward and may be understood as a confrontation between expectations and actualities. Rita Charon's work in this area is presented as an example. Existential phenomenology carefully describes concrete experience as it unfolds in the person's life. In existential health psychology, an existential phenomenological analysis would examine how an illness is lived and how their body is experienced throughout the course of the illness.

Keywords Qualitative research • Narrative medicine • Phenomenological psychology • Hermeneutic phenomenology

In order to examine the existential dimension of healthcare—the part that has been systematically ignored by medical science—a hermeneutic shift in methodological perspective is necessary. The necessary shift is from an abstract attitude to one of concretion. This is precisely the opposite of the shift effected by modern science.

© The Author(s) 2019
P. M. Whitehead, *Existential Health Psychology*,
https://doi.org/10.1007/978-3-030-21355-8_7

Concrete experience is what unfolds in the first person. This is what it is like to be you right at this moment—the undifferentiated flow of affective, temporal, spatial, and embodied modes of existence. This is your experience *before* it has been organized into objectifiable features *about* your experience. When your skin is flush with a fever, there is a concrete experience of this. You cannot *experience* the failure of thermoregulation. What you experience is a series of shifts in comfort within your environment. Five blankets are suddenly not adequate in managing the feverish chills. Your search for comfort includes a survey of possible relationships between yourself and your environment—whether it be making hot tea, donning a second sweater, or finding an extra blanket. Then suddenly your body erupts with heat as though you could plunge yourself headlong into a snowbank.

The concrete experience of a fever unfolds in this uncertain and multifaceted way. It does not, of course, only affect your temperature. It also affects your perception. The appeal of certain routines such as going to work, keeping social plans, and exercise have also changed. Familiar levels of patience, irritability, and interest have changed along with your diet. Moreover, these changes do not occur in any preset, generalized fashion, but only ever occur to a person within her world of meaningful relationships. To lump all of these together into symptoms of "fever" is to take up an abstract relationship to the concrete experience of discomfort.

That a body's temperature has risen 3° is a fact of medical science. It is an objective, publicly verifiable observation. The examples of discomfort can be subjectively reported, but these are for the most part private. They do not have the quality of public verifiability the way that a temperature, as measured by a thermometer, does.

Your temperature is not synonymous with your discomfort, either. You might go to the doctor's office and complain about your discomfort. An attending nurse might take your temperature, finding that it is 102°. You are diagnosed with a fever—you *have* a fever. The many concrete experiences of discomfort are translated into the abstract category of fever. Once (or if) you understand your experience this way—namely, that you *have* a fever—then you will have succeeded in making a hermeneutic shift *from* concrete *to* abstract. It is a very different way of relating to your experience. Instead of being personal and meaningful, these uncertain feelings of discomfort have been transformed into bits of evidence to be gathered by a modern scientific detective (not unlike the physician Arthur Conan Doyle). Instead of trying to understand the discomfort *as it is lived*, you have succeeded in taking the perspective of a detached third-person observer—exactly the way that medical scientists understand human existence. The goal in the practice of existential medicine is to reverse this shift.

Philosopher Don Ihde (2012) describes the hermeneutic shift brilliantly in his discussion about maps as an instance of human technology. A map is an abstraction of the land it represents. Indeed, it is an inert, two-dimensional representation of a three-dimensional, active, concrete world. To look down at this slip of paper (or glowing smartphone application) and know that "You are here" is to perform a hermeneutic shift in perspective with respect to your awareness of space and location. This shift is *from* concrete *to* abstract.

After finishing up a short road race in downtown Atlanta, a few friends and I were interested in finding a place to eat breakfast. We found ourselves on a sidewalk beside a six-lane road, surrounded by skyscrapers on three sides and a park on the fourth. Cars were whooshing past and we could still hear the race director calling out instructions to the runners who were still completing the race. I opened the map application on my smartphone and typed "breakfast" into the miniature search bar. There was a diner only two blocks away. Using the street signs as reference points, we were able to determine the direction needed to get to the diner. In this act, I transformed the active roads before me into little yellow lines on a map grid on the face of my glowing smartphone. I then transformed our location in concrete space and time into the generic, two-dimensional space on the map: "we are here, and we need to get to there." "There" was also an abstract location, a beige square marked with a blue dot beside the yellow line.

Whenever we use a map, we accomplish a hermeneutic shift from concrete to abstract. Once we get to our location, we hopefully shift back into concrete experience. However, it would be possible to live for a time within this world of abstractions, such as following along with what the online reviews suggest to order at the diner, eating the recommended well-balanced breakfast, and so forth.

The practice of modern science has also effected a hermeneutic shift from concrete to abstract. This shift has even been celebrated by child psychologist Jean Piaget as the highest level of thinking. For Piaget, the final cognitive developmental shift is from what he calls concrete operations to formal (abstract) operations. In the world of concrete operations, children explore the properties of things *as they are experienced*. This latter point captures the significance of the adjective "concrete" to describe the cognitive operations at this third stage of development. Big objects are big because they *seem* big. Heavy is reserved for objects that *seem* heavy. Abstract concepts like "infinite" and "probability" are impossible to understand because they cannot be experienced concretely. Infinite *seems* like something so vast that it could never be counted. Flipping a coin and having it land on heads *seems* less probable than having it land on tails when the last ten flips were heads. In order to achieve the fourth stage of cognitive development, children must deny their experience of the concrete qualities of the world in order to privilege these abstract qualities. They learn that a line segment that is one inch long has the same number of points on it than a line segment that extends infinitely (the answer for both is "infinite"). They learn that the Earth is always rotating and travels over 500 million miles every year, even though it *seems* like it is perfectly still. The person who succeeds in formal operations has learned to discredit her concrete experience, and to privilege logic and rationality.

In this same manner, people who have been trained in formal operations eventually learn to observe their own body as an object, even when this is in direct conflict with their experience. Rather than feel *their* skin's sense-giving properties as points of sensorial contact with the world, they begin to view their fingerprints the way that they have been characterized on television as uniquely identifying signatures useful for law enforcement. They cannot, of course, *see* this fingerprint without rotating their concrete finger in front of their eyes. Even still they do not see black lines on a white background, but a series of gestalt lines made out of white, black, red, and brown hues. They also learn that touch is so sensitive in the fingertips because of the dense collection of nerve cells that sit beneath a few layers of skin. In short, they learn to view the living body *through which* they experience their world as an object that may be viewed from the perspective of detached observer. *Leib* is exchanged for *Körper*.

The methods that are useful in existential medicine and existential health psychology are those that encourage this hermeneutic shift in the reverse: from abstract back to concrete. From here, the existential dimension of well-being can be examined in its concreteness and the *person* can be treated. These methods treat the human being in her existentiality. In so doing, they follow the methodological school of Wilhelm Dilthey known as "human science."

Wilhelm Dilthey and the Philosophy
of Human Science

It is difficult to imagine the use of the word "science" without also having in mind that practice of publicly verifiable analysis of the world in its objectivity. In order to imagine an alternative approach to modern science, you must first suspend what you understand as "science." Instead of "the generation of knowledge by way of the detached, third-person observation," think of science as "the generation of knowledge"—the definition it had in the nineteenth century. Now we can begin to think of a "human science" that does not equate a living person to a lump of human flesh on the examining table.

To begin with, the human scientist must recognize that the very factors of influence that affect her subject matter affect her as well. This is, in principle, very different from how we imagine the white-lab-coat-wearing physician in her examining room. The physician's mood need not interfere with the administration of a drug. The potency of a given drug is indifferent to the mood of the physician, but a person is not. If an irritated physician enters the examining room and begins the patient examination, an interaction has inevitably occurred—a human one. Variously, the patient will misinterpret the physician's irritation with something she may or may not have done as patient, or, following the lead of the physician's cool indifference, take herself to be like an anonymous patient history with certain biomedical properties. She might even leave the clinic with a pharmacy prescription that will be followed the way that she followed instructions to keep her Christmas Cactus from dying before the holidays were over.

The human scientist differs from the natural scientist in that the former's subject matter is necessarily personal. A geologist examines how pressure, temperature, and time come together to create limestone. The geologist herself is subject to the variables of pressure, temperature, and time, but these are not integral to her personality. The limestone does not exist the same way as the geologist does. In order to examine the substance of life, a new approach must be taken. Wilhelm Dilthey argued that the human sciences ought to be distinct from the natural sciences. "The expression of 'life,'" Dilthey (ND) tells us,

> denotes what is to everyone the most familiar and intimate, but at the same time the darkest and even most imponderable. ... One can describe it. One can elucidate its peculiar and characteristic traits. One can, as it were, inquire

after its tone, rhythm, and melody. But one cannot analyze it totally into all its factors, for it is not totally resolvable in this manner. What it is cannot be expressed in a simple formula or explanation. Thought cannot fully go behind life, for it is the expression of life. (Quoted in Polkinghorne 1983, p. 25)

Dilthey explains that human sciences must emphasize concrete experience as it is lived by people. Only in that manner can the human being be understood. This type of knowledge can be understood through the German word *verstehen*. *Verstehen* refers to a type of knowledge that is different from facts about things. *Verstehen* deals with the understanding of another person. We sometimes call such understanding empathy, because it has to do with trying to understand the meaning of an experience *from the vantage point of another person*.

Dealing with personal meaning is a difficult project. Experience is unimaginably thick, and it unfolds upon many horizons of meaning: a person's biography, how they view themselves, how they imagine others view them, where they see themselves going, how they are feeling, and so on (Merleau-Ponty 1962; Boss 1979; Condrau 1988). These horizons of meaning are not variables to be added to the bottom line of a ledger either: each contributes an undifferentiable element of the whole. The process of trying to understand this meaning is daunting. When faced with someone's concrete, unabstracted experience, we typically want to hide, because this makes us feel something concrete ourselves. The experience of the Other (person), taken fully as Other (person), demands of us our total presence, and we cannot help but be changed by the process (Buber 1962). This theme is developed further by American psychologist Jonathan Gibson (2017).

Human science emphasizes meaning, intention, and understanding. It involves getting in touch with your experience of vision, memory, athleticism, romance, problem solving, and so on. It is only *through* these ways of being in the world that an illness can ever be lived. This perspective recognizes that you are of the world—engaged in interrelationships with people, events, and things. You are not merely being manipulated and shaped by external forces. These words are not binary signs that are bombarding your brain and altering its chemistry and thereby altering you. They are words that may or may not be of significance to you. Words that you might grapple with, reject, or take up and apply in a unique way.

Two examples will be shared below in order to demonstrate human science methods that might be useful for examining the existential dimension of medicine. They are not intended to exhaust the potential of research along these lines, but in order to serve as an example of what is possible. The first is narrative medicine, and the second is existential phenomenology.

NARRATIVE MEDICINE: EXAMINING NARRATIVE STRUCTURES OF MEANING

Following the perception theory of the Berlin school, French phenomenologist Maurice Merleau-Ponty (1962) has argued that perception is always meaningful. That is to say, insofar as a perception registers at all, it is held together by a distinct and familiar fabric of meaning. Occasionally, we experience what he calls perceptions of ambiguity—perceptions that are unclear for a moment such that it seems like we are seeing nothing at all. Psychologists Jerome Bruner and Leo Postman (1949) have comically demonstrated this with their experiment with anomalous playing cards. Subjects were shown playing cards with impossible color—suit combinations such as a black four of hearts. In some cases, subjects reportedly stared blankly at the cards, unable to say anything about what it was they were seeing.

Perceptions are ambiguous when there is no familiar horizon upon which to understand them. Personal experiences that unfold like this leave you thinking "wait, what happened just then?" Even in such moments, a brief reflection will allow the seemingly disparate elements to cohere around a central meaning. This process is understood as constructing a narrative of meaning for an event. Narrative inquiry is a method where a researcher works alongside a subject to try to understand the familiar narrative around which their experiences cohere.

A stomachache never presents in a generic form, but always fits into a particular sequence of experiences. Having just eaten something outside of one's normal routine, the stomachache will seem like an indicator of nausea brought on with the unfamiliar food. If following a fistfight, then it will seem like a muscular contusion to the abdominal muscles. And there wouldn't be any notice of discomfort if engrossed in a movie or a conversation.

The significance of sequentiality grows when the medical problem includes severe trauma, such as damage to the spinal cord or brain, resulting in a substantial change to one's personality and normal routine. As such, one's post-injury self and routine must be reconciled with the pre-injury self and routine. Previous ways of being-in-the-world are no longer possible. Daily routine—getting out of bed, getting dressed, preparing food, taking care of oneself, interacting with others, engaging in the tasks of one's occupation—must be engaged in a wholly different capacity or as a different person. As such, rehabilitation is not just a process of rebuilding the muscular-skeletal system, but also requires a re-acquainting of an injured person with their new potentialities.

After a traumatic accident leaves a person paralyzed, a new narrative must be generated. Few able-bodied people imagine a narrative for their life wherein they have overcome the inability to use their legs. They have never had to wonder what it might be like to be unable to use their legs. For paraplegics, post-injury life will necessarily be different from pre-injury life. Therefore, a reconciliation must occur. The kinds of things that they used to be able to do easily and comfortably before their injury have now become difficult, uncomfortable, and even impossible. Before an injury left him paralyzed, my father was an athletic, active, and able-bodied man. Small chores around the house were simple, as was a trip to the grocery store. After his injury, these simple tasks became far more complicated—for him and for my family. Without developing a new narrative that appreciates the substantial nature of the change my father had undergone as a paraplegic, the trips to the grocery store would continue to present as a problem for him and for us.

In the 2018 Jefferson Lecture in the Humanities (October 18), sponsored by the National Endowment for the Humanities, Rita Charon describes the practice of narrative medicine as it unfolds in the examining room. Charon is a physician and literary scholar who has founded the Program in Narrative Medicine at Columbia University. In her lecture, Charon explains how she and her colleagues have been using techniques borrowed from the humanities for their practice of medicine— "reappropriating the body of the sciences who have kidnapped it" (np).

Charon outlines three movements of their approach: Attention, Representation, and Affiliation. Attention refers to the process of listening. Not simply listening for the facts about the patient history, but listening *to* the patient as she speaks. Charon compares this to the process of deep reading in the humanities, where every word and phrase is carefully examined within its context in order to get a deeper sense of their significance. What she describes sounds very much like Martin Buber's existential phenomenological analysis of the self-Other relationship. Buber explains how I can always take up one of two types of relationships with an Other: I can *be with* an Other in a dynamic and mutually transformative capacity, aware of the depth of their existence; or I can be *alongside* an Other, treating them more or less the way I might treat my cup of coffee—something I ignore until I am ready for another sip. Attending is the first kind of attentional awareness. The physician is immersed in the being and expression of her patient.

Representation is the next step and is a slight modification of the patient-history report. After collecting all of the useful medical details, Charon explains how she then turns the computer monitor and keyboard toward the patient, asking if anything has been left out. Patients are then free to see if they may have misstated some of their experiences, or if their doctor may have misunderstood. The process is not unlike the client-centered therapy of humanistic psychotherapist Carl Rogers. Rogers maintains that what is most helpful in therapy is not expert advice, but being heard, understood, and accepted. After a client has shared something, Rogers will describe what it is he has heard—checking back in with the client to see if he is on the right track. This also gives the client an opportunity to reevaluate what she has said, and maybe find that she has left something out. Like Rogers, Charon has found that this practice has opened up dimensions of the patient's life that were previously assumed to be unimportant, such as deaths, fears, goals, or motivations. These dimensions shed insight into the patient's experience of the illness.

Attention and Representation come together in the third and final movement of narrative medicine: Affiliation. In this movement, patient and provider come together to contemplate human finitude and the limits of medical science. The suffering of the patient is not a dependent variable to be influenced as an effect of an independent variable, but a burden that must be borne by the patient alone. Through this process of reflection, a transformation occurs—a transformation like the one described in Chap. 6. In a 2007 article on narrative medicine, Charon describes it as like the process of psychoanalysis, where each participant reflects on the transference and countertransference that emerges.

EXISTENTIAL PHENOMENOLOGY

While narrative analysis and narrative medicine seek to examine the *stories* through which patients understand their medical issues, existential phenomenology examines the *structure* of the experience of illness itself. Like narrative analysis, the method of existential phenomenology requires a hermeneutic shift *from* abstract *to* concrete. However, rather than look for a storyline, existential phenomenologists look for structures of meaning based on familiar existential modes of being. These modes were described at the end of Chap. 4; they are spatiality, temporality, embodiment, sociality, and mood. As articulated initially by German philosopher Martin Heidegger in his 1927 book *Sein und Seit*, these five modes comprise the *how* by which existence unfolds. Human being is always beholden to these five modes, and losing any one of them is profoundly disorienting.

Structure of Existence   Look at the chair, couch, bed, ottoman, or whatever it is that you are seated on as you read this. For the sake of discussion, let us say that it is a couch. The couch is there, beneath you. It has particular dimensions such as length, width, and height, and these allow it to be placed into a situational relationship with respect to other objects in the room. If it were facing the wall, and pushed right up against it, then it would not be easy to access as a place to sit, and harder still to sit on. Its situatedness with respect to the room allows it its functionality. It is an opening that makes sitting a possibility. You might even imagine that the couch has the quality of being-there-for-you, but this is not entirely correct. We already understand that an important aspect of its being-there-for-you is its placement within the room. The couch is only inviting to you as a place to sit insofar as it has been placed in a manner that allows it to be used as such, and this agency is denied the couch. Instead, we must understand that the couch has been placed-there-for-you (i.e., by another person).

The being of a person is fundamentally different from the being of a couch. These are things that are merely there. Things have objectifiable qualities such as extension and duration, hardness and softness. Objectifiable qualities do not belong to the couch but are comparisons (measurements) to other objects. To say that the couch is seven-feet long is to compare it to the king's feet: the couch is the length of seven royal feet, placed end to end. Its hardness/softness is understood only in comparison to the hardness/softness of other objects. To say that these qualities *belong to the couch* is an abstraction. The comparison necessarily happens outside of the object—that is, between couch and king. The system of measurement has become so standardized that it has become synonymous with what we mean by *real*.

To say that the couch is in the living room means that there is a couch object in an open space. By virtue of its dimensions, we might understand that the couch "takes up space" in the room, because physics tells us that there is a finite amount of volume allowed in any three-dimensional space, and only so many couches could fit in there. Human beings can also be understood as objects that take up space. There are international records for how many humans can be fit into the available space within a car or telephone booth. The piling of persons into a car is not for the sake of driving anywhere, as safe driving would certainly be out of the question. So too with the phone booth. But even in these circus conditions, human beings are not merely there, they are existing. Humans occupy space. "Occupying" is a gerund and suggests that some event is unfolding.

A couch is in a room. Gravity draws it toward the floor. For a human being, the couch can be an object that must be negotiated when walking through the room, but it is also an invitation: an opening to sit, to recline, to relax, or to rest. If you are looking for a place to rest for a moment, then the couch is not "in the way" nor is it "taking up space." In this situation, the couch provides space for resting. Even though the couch object is taking up space in the room, for the tired person the couch is an *addition*—it is extra rest-giving space.

The natural and behavioral sciences take as their subject of investigation the characteristics of object things. They can test the rest-giving capacity of a couch and the multitude of factors that interact with this relationship. While illustrative and insightful regarding the qualities of things, these methods do nothing to touch the quality of existence in human beings. This is where existential phenomenology comes in. Instead of dividing the human being into a body and mind, and subdividing these dimensions into countless subcategories of mind stuff and body stuff, existential phenomenology takes the unique qualities of a particular human being as its subject. The goal is not conceptualizing or classifying, but opening and describing. Working *with* (never *on* or *over*) one person at a time, the existential phenomenologist seeks to understand the structure of meaning of a person's existence.

It has become popular of late to describe the world of objects as if they exist in the same way that humans do. Such approaches have been called "object-oriented" and "speculative." As it stands, there is no way to investigate the being of objects in this manner without having humans speculate about what this might look like. Any conclusion, of course, would necessarily be human centric. I cannot know if the coffee table in the living room meaningfully occupies space on our rug the same way my wife does when she is doing yoga. I cannot know if the table stretches or focuses on breathing as she does. As such, existential phenomenology would not be a very insightful method for understanding coffee tables. Just as an existential analysis of a coffee table would be unhelpful for understanding the latter, so too would an experimental method be unhelpful for understanding the existential dimension of health. As it has been described above, health can only be understood in this manner.

Rather than abstract the existential unfolding of illness into bits of objective criteria to be manipulated by medical science, existential phenomenology examines the entire structure of an illness experience through each of these modes. An injury or illness does not affect a body, but a person. It affects their relationships, goals, and aspirations. In order to understand the significance of an injury or illness, the entire pre-injury personality must first be understood as Boss (1979) and Goldstein (1934/2000) remind us.

Clinical Research and Clinical Intervention To avoid treading into ethically uncertain territory, it is important to differentiate the role of the existential phenomenologist (and narrative medicine) from the role of the psychological therapist. To do so we must first differentiate the verbs "helping" from "understanding." Therapists are tasked with helping; researchers are tasked with understanding. Therapists intervene and thereby foreclose; researchers seek to understand and thereby open. It is worth recognizing that narrative medicine training includes analytic training—a form of clinical supervision. But one does not need to be clinically supervised to conduct research along these lines. This chapter is not about medical intervention, but about understanding.

A therapist is a state-licensed practitioner. The license certifies that the therapist has been duly educated in the diagnosis of state-recognized diseases, disorders, and illnesses, and has been duly trained in their state-sanctioned best practices of intervention. Therapists are educated and trained to work with diagnoses and interventions. As the state elects to change diagnostic criteria or interventional strategies, the therapists amend their practices accordingly.

Patients seek the help of a therapist when they believe that they have a particular and diagnosable problem. Something that might be objectified by medical science. If the credentialed therapist or clinician diagnoses their problem as such, then the intervention can begin. The intervention requires the transformation of the patient by the hand of the therapist—such as through a neurochemical agent (such as an antidepressant), cognitive practice (such as breathing or meditation), or bodily manipulation (such as a massage). In these interventions, the therapist is active while the patient is passive. The therapist is dictating the terms while the patient either is compliant and accepts them or is noncompliant and rejects them.

Insofar as she is trained in narrative inquiry or existential phenomenology, the qualitative researcher does not deal in diagnoses or interventions. The abstract diagnostic category by itself is unhelpful as it does nothing to illuminate a concrete experience of a problem. By shining light on only certain, state-approved symptoms of a particular disorder (and thereby casting a shadow on the non-state-approved elements of a person's experience of their life as a problem), a diagnosis can actually be counterproductive to the process of better understanding the transformation the person is undergoing. Furthermore, without a diagnosis, there is nothing to intervene against. There is no problem that can be understood as something *in addition* to the person's life. There is only the life of the person in question (the patient person, or person who is patient with his or her discomfort).

Interventions are other-directed. The therapist, from a privileged and state-certified perspective, intervenes on the life of the patient. The intervention necessarily has the quality of limitation. In an intervention, a space of possibility is being closed off. This brings us once again to Goldstein's (1934/2000) existential dimension inherent in all medical interventions. A patient either accepts greater suffering along with greater independence, or seeks a decrease in suffering (and a decrease in independence).

It is not the business of researchers to intervene, and they should reject any suggestion to do so. The researcher is interested in understanding the patient. Insofar as the topic is health, the researcher is tasked with understanding how health has become a problem for the person in question. That is to say, in which ways has their health become relevant to the patient at all.

The injury is not limited to the damaged tissue but extends to the entire life of the person. As Gadamer (1996) would say, one's well-being is damaged. Therefore, in order to understand the impact of an injury, we cannot look only at the tissue damage, but must look at the complete transformation of the personality that has been necessitated.

> The sick person is no longer simply identical with the person he or she was before. For the sick individual 'falls out' of things, has already fallen out of their normal place in life. But the individual who now lacks and misses something previously enjoyed still remains orientated towards returning to that former life. (p. 42)

The existential phenomenologist examines this particular "falling out" as a singular case of a phenomenon of a given injury. They begin with the personality before a patient's health became a problem for them, particularly those areas that have now presented as problems. For example, since the injury, the patient now has trouble working.

REFERENCES

Boss, M. (1979). *Existential foundations of medicine and psychology* (S. Conway & A. Cleaves, Trans.). New York: Jason Aronson.

Bruner, J. S., & Postman, L. (1949). On the perception of incongruity: A paradigm. *Journal of Personality, 18*(2), 206–223.

Buber, M. (1962). *I, Thou* (R. G. Smith, Trans., 2nd ed.). New York: Scribner.

Condrau, G. (1988). A seminar on Daseinsanalytic psychotherapy. *The Humanistic Psychologist, 16*(1), 101–129.

Gadamer, H. (1996). *The enigma of health: The art of healing in a scientific age* (J. Gaiger & N. Walker, Trans.). Stanford: Stanford University Press.

Gibson, J. (2017). A relational approach to suffering: A reappraisal of suffering in the helping relationship. *Journal of Humanistic Psychology, 57*(3), 281–300.

Goldstein, K. (2000). *The organism.* New York: Zone. (Original work published in 1934).

Ihde, D. (2012). *Experimental phenomenology: Multistabilities* (2nd ed.). Albany: SUNY Press.

Merleau-Ponty, M. (1962). *Phenomenology of perception* (C. Smith, Trans.). New York: The Humanities Press.

Polkinghorne, D. (1983). *Methodologies for the human sciences: Systems of inquiry.* Albany: SUNY Press.

CHAPTER 8

Post-Concussion Syndrome: An Exemplar

Abstract This chapter describes post-concussion syndrome (PCS) using the method of hermeneutic phenomenology. The analysis focuses on three cases of PCS: two National Collegiate Athletic Association Division I and II football players, and a college professor and amateur mountain climber. Each sufferer describes a change to his or her pre-injury personality and lifestyle, and a careful analysis of these stories demonstrates how PCS plays out along horizons of temporality, sociality, and embodiment.

Keywords Post-concussion syndrome • Traumatic brain injury • Hermeneutic phenomenology • Qualitative research

In order to demonstrate the significance of the hermeneutic shift with respect to healthcare that I described in the previous chapter, I will describe the consequences of doing so. The topic I have examined is the now-obsolete psychiatric condition once known as post-concussion syndrome (PCS). Like all psychiatric diagnoses listed in the *DSM*, PCS (which is no longer listed in the most recent version) is based entirely on subjective observations that a patient has about his or her condition. Also like all of the psychiatric diagnoses listed in the *DSM*, there is no way of corroborating whether or not a patient *has* or *does not have* the condition outside of his or her subjective reports. However, unlike the rest of the diagnoses listed in the *DSM*, PCS has been removed for its lack of corroborating evidence.

As its name indicates, PCS is a disorder that follows one or more concussions. The concussion is followed by a predictable series of immediate symptoms, which include loss of consciousness, dizziness, disorientation, headaches, fatigue, insomnia, trouble focusing, and so on. There are also measurable differences in neurological activity such as cerebral blood flow. These measurable changes are expected to continue for a short period following the minor traumatic brain injury (mTBI) before the patient's normal routine returns. In PCS, however, the normal routine does not resume, and patients continue to suffer from one or more of these symptoms for several months and sometimes years.

After the measurable neurological changes associated with mTBI have dissipated, there is no way of verifying whether or not a patient is legitimately suffering from PCS, or some other associated psychiatric condition such as anxiety. This is why the *DSM-V* has removed it from diagnostic consideration. Thus, instead of a legitimate psychiatric condition, PCS may be understood as a medically unexplained physical symptom (MUPS). MUPS are problems that seem to be physiological in origin, even though there are no identifying physiological markers. As a MUPS, PCS is in good company. Nearly 40% of medical complaints come from MUPS, including chronic pain, stomachaches, nausea, and dizziness (Slatman 2018). While my infrequent migraine headaches are debilitating to me, there is no way to prove to my wife that I am actually suffering and not, for example, performing an elaborate ruse to avoid running errands.

Even though they make up a substantial percentage of medical cases, MUPS cannot be treated by medical science as there is no objective measure for impairment or, if given treatment, improvement. In order to demonstrate effective treatment of chronic pain, for example, a physician must demonstrate the subjects report a lower level of pain after their course of treatment. But such subjective reports fall well short of the gold standard of medical science.

In place of PCS in the *DSM-V* you will find the diagnostic categories of acute stress disorder and neurocognitive disorder associated with TBI. The neurocognitive disorder is not diagnosed by a measurable change to the nervous system, but to the speed and accuracy with which the patient completes a neurocognitive inventory as conducted by a neuropsychiatrist. Acute stress disorder is a general category that fits a variety of symptoms that do not appropriately fall into any other available diagnosis. This general list of symptoms is found below. If these symptoms have continued for longer than a month, the diagnosis would change to post-traumatic stress disorder.

Because mTBI is common among contact-sports athletes, it would be worthwhile to consider the diagnosis of PCS followed by the National Collegiate Association of Athletics (NCAA)—this is the one supplied by the *International Classification of Diseases, 10th Edition.* The *ICD-10* allows a diagnosis of PCS to be made on the patient's subjective report of symptoms. Like the possible symptoms associated with acute stress disorder in the *DSM-V*, the symptoms of PCS in the *ICD-10* are vast:

Headache	Nervousness
Dizziness	Stress intolerance
Vertigo	Alcohol intolerance
Memory problems	Fear of permanent brain damage
Concentration problems	Malaise
Attention problems	Noise intolerance
Anxiety	Multitasking difficulty
Emotional or affective lability	Problems shifting focus
Fatigue	Apathy or lack of spontaneity
Depression	Decreased rhythmic accuracy
Insomnia	Decreased music-listening pleasure. (Boyd 2014, p. 117)

Notice how none of these symptoms can be corroborated objectively, but that each represents a substantial change to a person's way of living. Any one of them can be debilitating, interfering with, or inhibiting one's daily routine. That is to say, each symptom suggests a change to one's way of being. They are problems to health (where health is defined not as the absence of pathogens, but as one's well-being or being-well). In order to understand and appreciate the gravity of these symptoms, we must first understand what well-being looks like for the patient in question. What did a normal day look like? What were the qualities of normalcy and predictability that the patient had taken for granted?

To begin, the PCS patient must have suffered from a minor TBI event with or without a loss of consciousness. After this injury, there was a period of several days where the patient experienced amnesia, disorientation, nausea, and/or fatigue. Rather than return to their normal routine after this period, the patient continued to experience disrupting symptoms. This is the general structure of PCS from a phenomenological hermeneutic perspective.

There is plenty to consider in the experience of PCS without looking at changes to cortical tissue or cerebral blood-flow patterns. Indeed, finding any *thing* that has changed in the patient's cortex would do little to help us understand the change they have experienced in their life. Instead of looking inside the patient's body, we will look at the change to his or her existence: in what way has the patient changed? We could say that it is the patient's personality that has changed, but such a change would necessarily have to come by way of the patient's experience. Therefore, it would be redundant to also call this a change to the person *and* her personality. The many symptoms of PCS listed in the *ICD-10* can be understood as an estrangement a person experiences from his or her body (as well as the other four dimensions of existentiality).

INVESTIGATING PCS EXISTENTIALLY

Along with American psychologist Gary Senecal, I interviewed individuals who reported experiencing PCS. Two were NCAA football players who had suffered multiple concussions, and the third was a college professor who sustained a concussion when a climbing partner fell on top of her. Each participant experienced symptoms that continued for at least several months. Formal analyses and case studies have been written for publication elsewhere, but I would like to outline a few of the overarching themes of what we found during our investigation. When reviewing these themes, one quickly finds a departure from the conventional analysis of a medical problem, but one that nevertheless proves important for understanding and treating a medical condition.

The Temporal Component There was a temporal component of PCS that each of our participants came up against. It wasn't that their judgment of time had become impaired, but that their relationship between past, present, and future had changed based on the mTBI experience.

From the perspective of objectivity that medical science takes, time is that which is measured by a clock or watch. Duration becomes the fourth dimension within which physical objects can be found (along with length, width, and depth). The objective dimension of time is divided up into equal units, from seconds to decades. These units are understood to unfold in a linear fashion: from past to present to future. Events that unfold in the past cause events to unfold in the present, and these two combine to cause events to unfold in the future. But this is not how time is *lived*.

Existentially, time becomes temporality, which includes the experience of duration as well as the background meaning supplied by past, present, and future. Existentially, it is unhelpful to explain that 1 minute is exactly 60 seconds. Some minutes pass by so rapidly that you can hardly keep up with them; others seem to take an eternity. The minutes pass rapidly for one who has much to do, and slowly for one who is waiting for something to happen. Also from an existential vantage point, time does not always move in a linear manner from past to future. While the past can certainly influence the future, the future can also influence the past. This is essential in order to understand PCS as it was lived by our participants.

Past Affecting the Present Each of our participants recognized a change in the present that could be traced to the concussions experienced in the past. For Tyrese, he wished to avoid having to sit on the bench for a month as well as receiving special consideration with his classes. His decision making in the present was influenced by what had happened in the past. Hannah, the rock climber, became anxious whenever she thought about belaying another climber because of what had happened.

In these ways, the past may be found influencing and shaping the present of our participants. Because this is the way that temporality is handled by medical science—that is, past trauma leading to impairments—it is not surprising to find the experiences of fear, uncertainty, and anxiety that are traceable to past instances of mTBI.

Future Affecting the Present Another change is observable to the participants' experience of their future. The direction of past to future is not an unusual one for medical scientists to adopt. Smoking now can lead to lung cancer later on down the road. Such causal attributions for events that have never happened are quite common in medicine. But it is seldom recognized that what is happening in these situations is how the future is influencing the present. The fear of what *might* happen is enough to change the choices made now (such as quitting smoking).

Our participants demonstrated how a concern about the possible loss of future aspirations was enough to influence the decisions they made in the present. Such concern is a familiar one with those who suffer from anxiety. Neo-Freudian psychoanalyst Karen Horney (1991) said it best when she defined anxiety as the gap between the present and the future. The future is what you hope for. It is that toward which your actions are directed. Since the future can never be predicted perfectly, that leads to uncertainty. However, rather than experience the uncertainty *in the future*, which is where it belongs, anxious persons experience it in the present. Ironically, and as existential therapist Rollo May (2015) observed, this often inhibits a person's ability to achieve the future they desire. This is evident in a student who is worried about making a mistake and embarrassing himself during a class presentation. His preoccupation with not making any mistakes distracts him from the presentation, leading to mistakes.

After his first three concussions, Tyrese began to worry about what would happen down the road. The possible relationship between concussion injuries from contact sports and severe mental disorders became a popular media topic following the suicide of Hall of Fame cornerback Junior Seau. Seau had been well known for his positivity on and off of the field as well his support for his teammates. In short, he was the last name that came to mind as a candidate for depression. But two years after retiring, he took his life. In the years that followed, the media was abuzz about the long-lasting impact of contact sports and what could be done to mitigate against these problems. This could also be seen in the youth athletics programs, where it became customary for young athletes to be educated on the diagnosis, prognosis, and treatment of concussions. Many school systems, including the one attended by Tyrese, began to implement post-concussion protocols such as taking time off from schoolwork and taking a break from the sport. This meant that Tyrese did not only have to worry about the complications of an mTBI, but the *possible* long-term consequences of PCS as well. There was a growing concern that the *next* concussion would be the one that ruins the rest of his life. Instead of being able to give all of himself to the sport, focusing entirely on the current play, Tyrese had to overcome this fear of future damage that another concussion would cause. I suspect that this was why he began to describe his presence on the field as being rage filled, rather than the enjoyable spirit of competition. The rage was necessary to overcome the fear that had emerged.

Kyle's experience with PCS was similar to that of Tyrese. Kyle's parents had shared their concern with him about the possible long-lasting impact of his concussions. He described wanting to be a father someday, and how he wanted to be able to finish college and work a job as a professional. For Kyle, there was always the possibility that the next concussion would put his future at risk. Another concussion might erase the possibility of his marriage, his happiness with an occupation, and his children. Because these were things he was working toward in the present, their possible erasure was experienced in the present. His decision to stop playing football was based on the concern about his future. He was still perfectly capable of playing, but he was worried that he may not even be a choice were he to sustain a more serious concussion.

We could not, of course, *see* these impairments by looking at the participants' cerebral cortexes. But the temporal context nevertheless proves consequential for understanding how PCS is lived.

Another important context that is essential to understanding PCS is the influence of society. It is doubtful that our football players would have chosen to retire from their sport had the media attention not focused on the relationship between mTBI and the development of mental disorders. The widely publicized belief that contact sports would inevitably lead to violent mood swings and severe depression had filtered down into middle and high school athletics programs. Children who participated in sports are now taught about this relationship before their seasons begin, and parents learn about it on the news. This social consciousness about the ill effects of brain injury supplies an important background for understanding what a particular head injury means.

Rehabilitation When PCS is viewed existentially, the goal is to understand how the sufferer's life has changed. As we have seen with Goldstein earlier, this means trying to see how the impaired personality differs from the pre-injury personality. While this might include an examination of the body and nervous tissue, there does not appear to be any observable problem that neuropsychiatrists have been able to locate. This is why PCS is no longer listed in the *DSM-V*. But existential medicine and health psychology are not limited to the body the way that medical science is, so they can instead examine shifts of meaning that have occurred in the PCS patients.

The football players we interviewed each made the decision to retire from their sport. Given the level at which they were competing, this was a considerable change in lifestyle. Varsity athletics at the university level is very demanding and requires the highest degree of commitment and excellence. Courses are selected around the athletic schedule of games, practices, and meetings. Social lives are often dictated by proximity and comprise friendships with teammates, coaches, and fans. Finally, the personal investment required often means that identity and self-esteem are tied to the sport as well. Viewed by itself, the decision to retire from the central element of their life results in a serious change.

Instead of viewing rehabilitation as a bodily fix, where the body is nursed back to its pre-injury state, existential rehabilitation involves adapting to the changes to personality and lifestyle that have occurred. A paralysis patient will not be rehabilitated back to his or her pre-injury state. The specifics of the injury preclude this. What must happen is that patient learn how to organize his or her lifestyle anew in the wake of the injury. This will mean making changes to routines, relationships, expectations, and goals. In short, a new meaningful lifestyle must be *allowed to emerge*. While this should occur naturally, what often happens is that a person holds on to the pre-injury lifestyle that is no longer possible. Here they are continuously confronted with their limitations, always frustrated as a person *with an impairment*. This prevents them from seeing alternative avenues of growth and meaning.

Entirely on his own, Tyrese found a way to reorganize his life after retiring from football. The absence of his primary sport left a massive gap. The team was very much like a family, with mentorship from coaches and a brotherhood among teammates. The sport also resembled an occupation, as a scholarship covered tuition and living expenses. In order to rehabilitate, Tyrese had to fill these two gaps and in so doing develop his post-injury personality.

First, he was able to take a break from classes and move back home. This substantially limited the scope of his responsibilities, preventing him from becoming overwhelmed with the gaping hole left by retiring from football. This is a normal response to a catastrophic situation; one Goldstein has called a restriction of milieu. From there, Tyrese got a full-time job selling retail products that were associated with football. This allowed him to keep a place for football in his new lifestyle, rather than writing it out completely. His social life followed his new employment. By spending time with his new coworkers, he realized that he could have non-football-related things in common with others, and, by extension, develop relationships with others that were not based in his identity as a football player. Feeling more capable and confident, Tyrese returned to being a full-time student.

In short, Tyrese found a new routine to live by. He did not have to eliminate all aspects of his pre-injury personality and was able to find new ways to actualize those. No longer tormented by the possible foreclosure of his future, the depression he had been experiencing began to lift. Indeed, during the interview he was already brainstorming ways that he could begin helping other athletes—professional and collegiate combined—recover from career-ending injuries associated with mTBI.

References

Boyd, W. D. (2014). *Post-concussion syndrome: An evidence-based approach.* Aurora: XLIBRIS.

Horney, K. (1991). *Neurosis and human growth: The struggle towards self-realization.* New York: W.W. Norton & Co.

May, R. (2015). *The discovery of being.* New York: W.W. Norton & Co.

Slatman, J. (2018). Reclaiming embodiment in medically unexplained physical symptoms (MUPS). In K. Aho (Ed.), *Existential medicine* (pp. 101–114). Lanham: Rowman & Littlefield.

CHAPTER 9

Conclusion: Caring for the Human Being—An Outline for Applied Existential Health Psychology

Abstract The concluding chapter can be read as a stand-alone introduction to existential health psychology and supplies a summary of four changes in perspective which a healthcare worker can make that will allow her to view her patients in their existentiality, thereby finding what was in their blind-spot. These are treating the *how* and not the what; understanding the illness in addition to the disease; treating the person and not the disease; and viewing the patient person in his or her Otherness, using the relational phenomenology of Martin Buber.

Keywords Medical providers • Medical practice • Nursing •
Phenomenology of nursing • Existential medicine • Martin Buber

This final, concluding chapter is designed to accomplish two tasks: first, it is intended to draw the preceding chapters together and bring them to a meaningful closure and, second, it is intended to be a stand-alone guide for those in the helping professions who wish to apply the insights of this book to their work with patient persons.

To begin, I will remind the reader why I have opted to refer to the consumer of medicine as a "patient person" rather than the more common term "patient" or, as has become popular in psychology, "client." When referring to a person as a patient, their unique and singular identity becomes replaced with their medical identity. It begins with the assumption

© The Author(s) 2019
P. M. Whitehead, *Existential Health Psychology*,
https://doi.org/10.1007/978-3-030-21355-8_9

that the only thing that matters about this person is that he or she has a virus, infection, or injury. You might even imagine a medical waiting room filled with damaged and diseased bodies, or as an anonymous collection of medical histories.

The term "patient" was not originally intended to be a noun in this manner, but an adjective. As an example of patient in the adjective form: kindergarten teachers are *patient* with young children. In this manner, we can understand that, medically speaking, a person is patient with his or her suffering. As such, they are patient persons, and they have come to you for assistance with this suffering.

Before getting into the brief overview of the chapters that have preceded this, and a subsequent presentation of four suggestions for providers, a few words must be shared about what I am *not* suggesting. I am not suggesting that we give up on the contemporary practice of medicine, and I am not suggesting that we throw away the evidence-based practices that have been carefully developed over many decades. I am not suggesting that we be skeptical of the practice *or* the practitioners of medicine. What I am suggesting is that something important is being left out of this mainstream medical practice, something personal and meaningful: the human quality of existence.[1]

The quality of patient care I intend to describe may be demonstrated by the medical experiences of two philosophers—one in the UK and the other in Florida. With the latter, all of his expertise in philosophy of medicine did not prepare Kevin Aho (2018) for the experience that he would have of being medicalized after a heart attack. His attending physicians and their staff treated his body as though it was a mere lump of matter with a broken pump. They treated him as a thing, a *what*. Probabilities of mortality/recovery were rattled off as though these did not have profound implications about his identities as a husband, friend, mentor, or colleague. As he experienced it, the interventions were directed at his inert, corporeal body—the lumped mass lying awkwardly on the hospital bed. There was no interaction with him—Aho-the-

---

[1] Incidentally, if I were to be speaking to a group of clinical psychologists and psychiatrists, then I *would* be advocating that we throw away evidence-based practices as they have been carried out in bad faith, with the hopeful expectation that psychology and psychiatry might actually be medicine. In so doing, psychology and psychiatry have turned their back on the problem of human suffering which cannot be medicalized.

person. One evening, he had just been given the diagnosis of ventricular tachycardia, which came with a particular probability of sudden death. He was to be fitted with a pacemaker. He describes this as a particularly dark moment. That is—until an evening nurse recognized something familiar in his eyes, something personal: confusion and fear. She saw *him*. She had received a similar diagnosis years before and described her own personal bout with the depression that followed. She let him touch the scar from her surgery. What she was doing cannot be classified as medicine—at least not in the mainstream, modern medical sense. What she shared with him was not in her job description and likely would not lead to a promotion or raise. If anything, she may have been sanctioned for this. Of this, and another personal connection had with an intensive care nurse, Aho writes: "each of these disclosures provided the recognition I desperately needed... to express and make sense of my shattered identity" (np).

Martin Kusch was a professor of philosophy of science at Cambridge when he went in for a routine dental procedure. A root canal became a tooth extraction, which became the extraction of two more teeth, and these were accompanied by severe chronic pain for a number of years. Kusch (Kusch and Ratcliffe 2018) describes his experience of being passed around from specialist to specialist, each offering a critique of the previous specialist and recommending their own course of treatment. The medications piled up, the procedures wore on, but the pain persisted. He found the experience to be a dehumanizing, disempowering, and deeply hopeless one. He eventually left the health management consortium that had been passing him around like an Old Maid card, and gave up on the idea of pain *cure*, looking instead to pain *management*. In sum, he took his well-being into his own hands instead of waiting for it to be a good that was the unique domain of specialized medical practice. He began to view his life in optimistic terms and experienced some of the lowest subjective levels of pain he had in years.

These stories came from philosophers, but I imagine that you will be able to think of similar stories told by people in your own life—perhaps even yourself. These are stories that demonstrate that medical *treatment* is not just a good or service, but deals with the way you and I *treat* one another as human beings.

ONE BODY OR TWO? *LEIB* AND *KÖRPER*

In the brief summary of the two vignettes I have just shared, I referred to the body in two very different ways. Each of these indicates a different way of relating to our bodies. In English, we just have the one word—"body." This word refers to the objective lump of tissue and bone *and* the necessary vehicle through which our experiences unfold (and which we refer to as our*selves*).

The first we call our corporeal or physical bodies. They are the bodies with definite measurements: so many inches, pounds, and so forth. Because they can only be understood in terms of these dimensions, the corporeal bodies are also the ones of science and, by extension, the bodies of medicine (since modern medicine is synonymous with medical science). We are referring to our corporeal bodies when we say things like: "I have fractured my tibia" or "my peroneal tendon is inflamed." In German, there is a single word that refers to the body this way: *körper*.

The second we call our lived bodies. These are the bodies through which we experience the world. Corporeal bodies may be poked, pricked, and palpated, but it is only through the *lived body* that you or I may touch another person (so as to poke, prick, or palpate them). The lived body is active and expressive. Were you to touch another person, perhaps the shoulder of a frightened child, you would not say "my hand has come into contact with your shoulder." Instead, you would say, I am *consoling* you. Lived bodies—human beings—can do that. The latter is a meaningful way of relating between persons; it is a way of self-expression. In German, the word *Leib* (living) is used to refer to this conception of the body.

The French existentialist author Jean-Paul Sartre has a helpful example comparing these two ways of understanding the body, which I will paraphrase for the purposes of this discussion. He is seated on the medical examination table just before an operation on his leg. The leg *is* him—that is to say, it is not just his leg that will be subjected to surgery, but *he* will be undergoing the trauma of surgery. This would be to assume that the surgical procedure on his leg will not affect his post-procedure metabolism, diet, mobility, and scope of activities. *He* will be affected. But as he sits on the table, he realizes that he can relate to his leg the same way that the doctors do. He can observe and point to his own leg the way he might point to or observe the leg of a patient person across the room, or on the television screen. With his fingers, he can trace the dotted line where the incision will go. *So you will make a two-inch incision laterally from the base of the patella*...and so on. This is his leg-as-object.

Can you guess which body has become the subject matter of modern medicine? Indeed, it is the corporeal body—*körper*. But after introducing both, it is peculiar that the discipline of medicine has taken as its subject matter the lifeless, inert, and abstracted body. Modern medicine, insofar as it is founded in evidence-based scientific practice, neglects the person *that exists through his or her body*. Existential medicine (Aho 2018) and existential health psychology aim at addressing this neglect (and hopefully you will too).

Health

Health has been treated as a scientific *effect*—that is, a measurable dependent variable—for so long that it has become difficult to define what it is *without* calling it the result of medical intervention.

Here's the number one answer I get when I ask my college students to define health: "Health is the absence of disease." This situates health within the specific early twentieth-century pathogenic model of treatment: locating and eliminating a virus, bacterial infection, or otherwise. But what is *restored* when one's health is restored. It certainly cannot be their lack of disease-ness.

French hermeneutic philosopher Hans Georg Gadamer attempts to resolve this riddle in his book *The Enigma of Health* (1996). He explains that health is so difficult to define *because it is precisely that state in which one is unconcerned with one's health*. You and I are healthy insofar as "health" is the furthest thing from our mind. If we are aware of, or actively seeking treatment for our health, it is only *then* that we are unhealthy. Well-being, then, could be understood as a state in which a person is able to go about their normal, personal, and meaningful life routine without inhibition or suffering.

Consider: is ankle pain a health concern? Were we to look at this from the pathogenic medical perspective, which states that health is the absence of disease, then we would begin by looking for signs of a pathogen in the ankle: swollen tendons, damaged tissue, bone spurs, and so on. Surgery could be scheduled to correct any of these hypothetical issues. However, were we to look at it with the conception of health as it is described by Gadamer, then we must first try to understand the ankle pain *within the context of the patient person's life*. Ankle pain does not belong to the ankle, but it is a change in the person's normal activities. As a long-distance runner, it is not unusual to experience ankle pain after a 20-mile run. Within that context, a bit of hobbling around would not stand out as problematic, or as a problem to solve. However, were I to experience the same ankle-pain-sensation after only two miles, I would begin to be concerned.

As you can see, "normal" ankle pain can only be understood within the context of the person who is experiencing it: that which is normal to him or her. It can only be understood through instances of difficulty walking from one room to another, or comfortably throughout the grocery store, where "comfortably" is defined as the routine manner by which this typically happens.

Unfortunately, "normal" means something entirely different when dealing with statistical distributions—the kind of distributions that are useful for analyzing enormous medical trials. To the latter, normal are those occurrences that land within +/− a single standard deviation from the mean in any population. Normal becomes standardized within a population. Similarly, health has become standardized.

Increasingly, health has become something you and I can work at. We can do healthy activities, eat healthy meals, and participate in healthy relationships. More and more aspects of our lives are recruited in service to our health. As you can see, this is the opposite of health as it has been defined by Gadamer, above. Following the late American psychiatrist Thomas Szasz (2012), I have called this process medicalization.

MEDICALIZATION

Medical interventions were once required only when diseases were present. A runny nose or a week of lethargy were understood to be within the range of normal human experience, but bouts of coughing with an elevated body temperature required treatment. In the last 70 years, treatments have become a way of life. Now "treatments" are routinely prescribed when there is nothing wrong. In the name of preventative medicine, health has become a problem for everyone. It is in this way that medicalization has insinuated itself into our personal lives.

More and more dimensions of life are seen through the glass of medicalization. We are taught to be ever vigilant against stress, the boogeyman of holistic medicine. "Chill out, bruh," we are told.

As they become increasingly medicalized, our lives begin to look less and less familiar to us. It becomes more common to refer to our own experiences through the processes of medicalization.

Four Steps for Viewing What Is in the Blind-spot

What I am suggesting is an antidote to medicalization—a method of balancing treatment of bodies (*körper*) with treatment of the person (and their living bodies; *leib*).

Rejecting medicalization is not synonymous with rejecting medicine. Medicine is as much an art as a science, as Gadamer (and Philippe Pinel) has argued. The art of patient care—a noun I find exceedingly appropriate—begins with remembering this subject matter.

The following are suggestions—not for specific actions, but for a change of mentality. I cannot tell you how to relate to the patient persons under your care, because this would result in imitation and mimicry. There would be dozens of providers pretending to treat their patients like human beings. However, once you begin to take them seriously, and relate to them as human beings, then the "what this looks like" will follow.

1. **Treat the *how*, not the *what*.** You do not have a cancer patient, you have a traumatized person whose anticipated future, and possibly present, has just been forever changed. This is not a diagnosis thing or a patient thing. It isn't a *what*. But it also wouldn't be accurate to refer to her as a *who*, because any identity, spoken by itself, becomes an abstraction of the living person before you. Instead, we can only understand her as a process—as a *how* (Aho 2018; Groth 2016).

Modern medicine deals with the *what*. It computes the lists of presenting symptoms and narrows down the diagnostic possibilities. It includes the procedures for taking tissue biopsies and examining them under a microscope. It includes the protocols for administering drug treatments or for setting broken bones. These may deal with the patient person's hip, now sore from the biopsy-needle entry, but they do not deal with the patient person.

The patient-care literature may remind providers to be mindful of the *who*. This, too, misses the point I am trying to make. It may be the case that your patient is a mother. This *means* something different to me than it does to you. "Mother" may be a more helpful noun than "woman," but it says nothing of this person's relationship with her children, or her experience of being a mother. Moreover, it does nothing to illustrate precisely *how* this person's illness has transformed her identity as a mother—much less any additional nouns that may also be useful in identifying her.

To repeat: your patient is not (only) a what *or* a who but also a how. The latter is where I am asking you to focus. This will hopefully be made clearer in the suggestions that follow.

2. **Illness, not disease.** The next shift in perspective I am suggesting here is to think of patients in terms of *illnesses* and not *pathologies* or *diseases*. This may sound like a meaningless request to replace one term with its synonym, but I have in mind two very different concepts.

"Disease" is a medical term that refers to the verified presence of a pathogen within an organism. Until it is corroborated by a medical specialist, there is no disease. If I began to experience stomach pains and nausea, I might think that I have pancreatitis. Were I to go to a provider complaining of these pains, I would not be treated for pancreatitis until a CT scan is run and the inflammation is seen on the wall of my pancreas. It is only at this point that I could be understood to *have* pancreatitis.

I don't *feel* pancreatitis, of course, what I feel are the pains and tightness somewhere around the area I understand my stomach to be. In his book *Absent Body*, philosopher and physician Drew Leder (1990) demonstrates many times over how poor we are at identifying sensations within our bodies. Is so-called stomach pain coming from the stomach, esophagus, pancreas, liver, or gall bladder? Or maybe it is in my abdominal wall. To be able to discriminate between each of these organs would require that we take an objective, third-person vantage point and view our body as an object (*körper*).

"Illness," on the other hand, refers to the singular suffering that a patient endures throughout the duration of a given problem. In a toothache, the illness would refer to the aching of the jaw that makes it difficult to chew, drink cold or hot beverages, and sometimes sleep. While an infection might be present within the tooth, a person cannot *feel* this—what she feels is a dull ache or sometimes shooting pain that is disruptive to how she is feeling. In an illness of any kind, the way of being for a person has become upset. Therefore, in order to understand an illness, you must first understand the person who is ill.

3. **Treat not the disease that has a person, but the person who is ill.** "Care more particularly for the individual patient than for the especial features of the disease" (in Bean and Bean 1961, p. 181). These are the famous words of William Osler (1849–1919), co-founder of the Johns Hopkins School of Medicine. For Osler, these words ought to guide all medical practice.

As defined above, it must be understood that an illness cannot be treated. Treatment can be administered to a body—a pancreas or tooth, but an illness refers to a change to a person's way of being. This patient person is not just a body, but a mother or father, a colleague, a friend, and professional, and has a set of unique and singular habits and hobbies with which he or she goes about his or her life. In illness, these rhythms have changed. Maybe they are more tired than normal. They don't *have* fatigue per se, but they may find themselves less patient with their children or coworkers. Each of these conditions can only be understood *through the manner by which they have transformed the patient person's ways of being.*

German neuropsychiatrist Kurt Goldstein (1878–1965), who gave psychologists the term "self-actualization," describes it this way: when trying to understand a particular condition or defect, it is not enough to focus only on the presenting symptoms. "Rather, it is imperative to consider the entire premorbid personality of the patient and his transformation by irreparable changes" (2000, p. 340).

It is interesting to see this shift in perspective already cropping up in the medical field.[2] For example, NPR in 2014 featured an article[3] by physician Leana Wen who describes the importance of being sensitive to the experience of the patient during treatment, and not just being focused on the affected body. She demonstrates this by describing the same event—a cardiac catheterization—from two different perspectives: that of the emergency room providers who viewed it as a textbook success, and that of the patient who filed a complaint a few days later. Also, proposals are being made in a variety of branches of medicine, for a more patient-centered approach, called "patient-centered care" (Morse 2016).

4. **Caring for an Other**. By putting the three previous suggestions together, we arrive at the fourth. The patient person is not a disordered body, she is not a heart pump, and she is not a nervous system; she is an Other (capital "O"). The relation you and I share with an Other is a primary one, because he or she also exists.

In his book *I and Thou*, Hebrew philosopher Martin Buber (1878–1965) describes two possible relationships we can share with the people we

---

[2] It is one I might expect to find within my own field of humanistic psychology, but by and large the latter have remained steadfast in their allegiance to the American Psychological Association. The latter is a proponent of the biomedical model of mental disorders.

[3] https://www.npr.org/sections/health-shots/2014/06/25/324005981/heart-of-the-matter-treating-the-disease-instead-of-the-person

encounter: the "I-Thou" relation, and the "I-it" relation. Beginning with the latter, we relate to another person as a thing. This is precisely what we do when we poke, prick, and palpate him or her. We may do this to measure pulse or collect a blood sample, but what we are dealing with is an object. Indeed, we call this type of data gathering "objective."

What Buber calls the "primary relationship" is the I-Thou relation, which may only be understood as a relation of mutuality. He explains, "The [Other] is no impression, no play of my imagination, no value depending on my Mood; but it is bodied over against me and has to do with me, as I with it—only in a different way" (1962, p. 8). Within this relation, there is no clear demarcation between self and Other. Your way of being (e.g. mood or temporality) draws forth something from the Other, just as she draws forth something in you. Interactions with a person who is anxious are likely to set your teeth on edge, just as an interaction with a person who is calm is likely to have a calming effect. Such a relation is dynamic, and oriented toward the future—that which is currently unfolding.

However, as soon as we say "let us look at your leg" or whatever the case may be, we introduce a gap between self and Other and take an I-it relationship to them. This is the subject-object relationship. In medicine, it is the unequal power distribution of doctor-patient, where the patient is the object being examined. There is no longer any reciprocity to the relationship. There is no interaction, and no exchange of meaning. "The barrier between subject and object has been set up. The primary word *I-It*, the word of separation, has been spoken" (p. 23).

The *I-It* relationship is a perspective that is foreign to human being: it negates our personal experience. It is an ideal of modern science, but it has gained power as a sort of God's-eye view of the world: seeing reality as it *actually* is, free from human error. It is ironic that the God's-eye view is the one that ignores that which is most deeply human.

It is only in treating the patient person as an Other—one who is always already engaged in a personal, reciprocal relationship with you—that you can experience the social dimension of existence—*Mitsein* or being-with-Others. This dissolves the over-and-above power relation, making it a human-human interaction.

REFERENCES

Aho, K. (2018). Chapter 11. Notes from a heart-attack: A phenomenology of an altered body. In C. Falke & E. Eriksen (Eds.), *Phenomenology of the broken body.* London: Routledge.

Bean, R. B., & Bean, W. B. (1961). *Sir William Osler: Aphorisms from his bedside teachings and writings* (p. 93). Springfield: Charles C. Thomas.

Buber, M. (1962). *I and Thou* (R. G. Smith, Trans.). New York: Scribner.

Gadamer, H. (1996). *The enigma of health: The art of healing in a scientific age* (J. Gaiger & N. Walker, Trans.). Stanford: Stanford University Press.

Goldstein, K. (2000). *The organism.* New York: Zone. (Original work published in 1934).

Groth, M. (2016). *After psychotherapy: Essays and thoughts on existential therapy.* New York: ENI Press.

Kusch, M., & Ratcliffe, M. (2018). The world of chronic pain: A dialog. In K. Aho (Ed.), *Existential medicine* (pp. 61–80). Lanham: Rowman & Littlefield.

Leder, D. (1990). *Absent body.* Chicago: University of Chicago Press.

Morse, J. (2016). *Qualitative health research: Creating a new discipline.* New York: Routledge.

Szasz, T. (2012). *Medicalization of everyday life: Selected essays.* Syracuse: Syracuse University Press.

REFERENCES

Aho, K. (2008a). Medicalizing mental health: A phenomenological alternative. *The Journal of Medical Humanities.* https://doi.org/10.1007/s10912-008-9065-1.

Aho, K. (2008b). Rethinking the psychopathology of depression: Existentialism, Buddhism, and the aims of philosophical counseling. *Philosophical Practice, 3*(1), 207–218.

Aho, K. (2017). A hermeneutics of the body and place in health and illness. *Place, Space, and Hermeneutics, 5,* 115–126.

Aho, K. (2018a). Existential medicine: Heidegger and the lessons from Zollikon. In K. Aho (Ed.), *Existential medicine* (pp. xi–xxiv). Lanham: Rowman & Littlefield.

Aho, K. (2018b). Neurasthenia revisited: On medically unexplained syndromes and the value of hermeneutic medicine. *Journal of Applied Hermeneutics, 6,* 1–14.

Aho, K. (2018c). Temporal experience in anxiety: Embodiment, selfhood, and the collapse of meaning. *Phenomenology and the Cognitive Sciences.* https://doi.org/10.1007/s11097-018-9559-x.

Aho, K. (2018d). Chapter 11. Notes from a heart-attack: A phenomenology of an altered body. In C. Falke & E. Eriksen (Eds.), *Phenomenology of the broken body.* London: Routledge.

Aho, K., & Guignon, C. (2011). Medicalized psychiatry and the talking cure: A hermeneutic intervention. *Human Studies.* https://doi.org/10.1007/s10746-011-9192-y.

Allan, R., & Fisher, J. (2011). *Heart and mind: The practice of cardiac psychology.* Washington: APA Press.

© The Author(s) 2019
P. M. Whitehead, *Existential Health Psychology,*
https://doi.org/10.1007/978-3-030-21355-8

American Psychiatric Association. (2013). *Diagnostic and statistical manual of mental disorders* (5th ed.). Washington, DC: APA.

Bean, R. B., & Bean, W. B. (1961). *Sir William Osler: Aphorisms from his bedside teachings and writings* (p. 93). Springfield: Charles C. Thomas.

Boss, M. (1979). *Existential foundations of medicine and psychology* (S. Conway & A. Cleaves, Trans.). New York: Jason Aronson.

Boss, M. (1988). Recent considerations in daseinsanalysis. *The Humanistic Psychologist, 16*(1), 58–74.

Boyd, W. D. (2014). *Post-concussion syndrome: An evidence-based approach.* Aurora: XLIBRIS.

Bruner, J. S., & Postman, L. (1949). On the perception of incongruity: A paradigm. *Journal of Personality, 18*(2), 206–223.

Buber, M. (1962). *I, Thou* (R. G. Smith, Trans., 2nd ed.). New York: Scribner.

Bugental, J. (1962). Humanistic psychology: A new breakthrough. *American Psychologist, 18*, 563–567.

Canguilhem, G. (1991). *The normal and the pathological* (C. R. Fawcett, Trans.). New York: ZONE Books.

Caruso, G. D., & Flanagan, O. (2018). *Neuroexistentialism: Meaning, morals, & purpose in the age of neuroscience.* Cambridge, MA: Harvard University Press.

Charon, R. (2018). *Keynote address.* Washington, DC: National Endowment of the Humanities.

Condrau, G. (1988). A seminar on Daseinsanalytic psychotherapy. *The Humanistic Psychologist, 16*(1), 101–129.

Cox, D., & Jones, R. P. (2017, November). *Searching for spirituality in the U.S.: A new look at spiritual but not religious.* Public Religion Research Institute. https://www.prri.org/research/religiosity-and-spirituality-in-america/. Accessed 20 Mar 2018.

Craig, E. (1988). Encounter with Medard Boss. *The Humanistic Psychologist, 16*(1), 25–57.

Craig, E. (1993). Remembering Medard Boss. *The Humanistic Psychologist, 21*(3), 258–276.

Erikson, E. (1994). *Identity and the life-cycle.* New York: Norton.

Freud, S. (1913). *The interpretation of dreams* (3rd ed., A. A. Brill, Trans.). New York: Macmillan.

Freud, S. (1914). *The psychopathology of everyday life* (A. A. Brill, Trans.). London: T. Fisher Unwin.

Gadamer, H. (1996). *The enigma of health: The art of healing in a scientific age* (J. Gaiger & N. Walker, Trans.). Stanford: Stanford University Press.

Gendlin, E. (2009). What first and third person processes really are. *Journal of Consciousness Studies, 16*, 33–62.

Gendlin, E., & Johnson, D. H. (2004). *Proposal for an international group for a first-person science.* New York: The Focusing Institute.

Gibson, J. (2017). A relational approach to suffering: A reappraisal of suffering in the helping relationship. *Journal of Humanistic Psychology, 57*(3), 281–300.

Goldberg, G., & Whitehead, P. (2017, October 25–28). The legacy of Kurt Goldstein: Person-centered healthcare, holistic biology, and biosemiotics in rehabilitation. In *American Congress of Rehabilitation Medicine national conference*, Atlanta.

Goldstein, K. (2000). *The organism.* New York: Zone. (Original work published in 1934).

Groth, M. (2016). *After psychotherapy: Essays and thoughts on existential therapy.* New York: ENI Press.

Healy, D. (2012). *Pharmageddon.* Los Angeles: University of California Press.

Heidegger, M. (2001). *Zollikon seminars: Protocols—Conversations—Letters* (M. Boss, Ed., and F. Mayr & R. Askay, Trans.). Evanston: Northwestern University Press.

Heidegger, M. (2008). *Being and time* (J. Macquarrie & E. Robinson, Trans.). New York: Harper Perennial. (Original translation published in 1962).

Horney, K. (1991). *Neurosis and human growth: The struggle towards self-realization.* New York: W.W. Norton & Co.

Ihde, D. (2012). *Experimental phenomenology: Multistabilities* (2nd ed.). Albany: SUNY Press.

James, W. (1909). *The meaning of truth.* New York: Dover Publications.

Kleinman, A. (1988). *Illness narratives: Suffering, healing, and the human condition.* New York: Basic Books.

Kusch, M., & Ratcliffe, M. (2018). The world of chronic pain: A dialog. In K. Aho (Ed.), *Existential medicine* (pp. 61–80). Lanham: Rowman & Littlefield.

Leder, D. (1990). *Absent body.* Chicago: University of Chicago Press.

Levinas, E. (1969). *Totality and infinity* (A. Lingis, Trans.). Evanston: Northwestern.

May, R. (2015). *The discovery of being.* New York: W.W. Norton & Co.

Merleau-Ponty, M. (1962). *Phenomenology of perception* (C. Smith, Trans.). New York: The Humanities Press.

Morse, J. (2016). *Qualitative health research: Creating a new discipline.* New York: Routledge.

National Institute of Diabetes and Digestive and Kidney Diseases. (2014). *Prevalence of overweight, obesity, and extreme obesity among adults: United States, trends 1960–1962 through 2013–2014.*

Olbert, C., & Gala, G. J. (2015). Supervenience and psychiatry: Are mental disorders brain disorders? *Journal of Theoretical and Philosophical Psychology, 35*(4), 203–219.

Polkinghorne, D. (1983). *Methodologies for the human sciences: Systems of inquiry.* Albany: SUNY Press.

Rogers, C. (1961). *On becoming a person: A therapist's view of psychotherapy.* New York: Houghton Mifflin.

Roser, M. (2018). Child and infant mortality. *Our World in Data*. https://ourworldindata.org/child-mortality

Russell, B. (2009). *Human knowledge: Its scope and its limits*. New York: Routledge. (Original work published in 1948).

Sartre, J. (1989). Existentialism is a humanism. In W. Kaufmann (Ed.), *Existentialism from Dostoevsky to Sartre* (P. Mairet, Trans.). New York: Meridian Publishing Company.

Slatman, J. (2018). Reclaiming embodiment in medically unexplained physical symptoms (MUPS). In K. Aho (Ed.), *Existential medicine* (pp. 101–114). Lanham: Rowman & Littlefield.

Szasz, T. (2008). *Psychiatry: The science of lies*. Syracuse: Syracuse University Press.

Szasz, T. (2010). *The myth of mental illness: Foundations of a theory of personal conduct*. New York: Harper Perennial.

Szasz, T. (2012). *Medicalization of everyday life: Selected essays*. Syracuse: Syracuse University Press.

Watson, J. (1913). Psychology as a behaviorist views it. *Psychological Review, 20*, 158–177.

Whitehead, A. N. (1920). *The concept of nature: The Tarner lectures delivered to Trinity College*. CreateSpace Publishing.

Whitehead, P. (2017). Goldstein's self-actualization: A biosemiotic view. *The Humanistic Psychologist, 45*(1), 71–83.

Wundt, W. (1896). *Gundriss der psychologie*. Leipzig: Wilhelm Engelmann.

Index[1]

[1] Note: Page numbers followed by 'n' refer to notes.

© The Author(s) 2019
P. M. Whitehead, *Existential Health Psychology*,
https://doi.org/10.1007/978-3-030-21355-8

CPSIA information can be obtained
at www.ICGtesting.com
Printed in the USA
LVHW081100180819
628039LV00014B/699/P